EVIDENCE-BASED TREATMENT PLANNING FOR SOCIAL ANXIETY DISORDER

DVD FACILITATOR'S GUIDE

TIMOTHY J. BRUCE

AND

ARTHUR E. JONGSMA, JR.

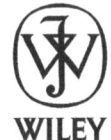

WILEY

John Wiley & Sons, Inc.

Contents

Introduction

This Facilitator *Guide* is designed to help you lead an educational training session in empirically informed treatment planning. It is to be used in conjunction with the DVD and its *Companion Workbook*. The Guide walks you through the process of delivering a training session.

The training session should be conducted in a comfortable room, where participants can read and write in their workbooks. A DVD player and monitor are required.

Organization

In this *Guide*, you will find in each chapter:

➤ Chapter review questions and answers
➤ Chapter review test questions and answers
➤ Talking points, this feature presents an optional question with a highlighted point or points to include in the discussion
➤ Therapeutic homework assignments
➤ Chapter references

In appropriate chapters, the references are divided into those for *empirical support*, those for *clinical resources*, and those for *bibliotherapy resources*. The empirical support references are selected studies or reviews of the empirical work supporting the efficacy of the treatments discussed in the chapter. The clinical resources are books, manuals, or other resources for clinicians that describe the application, or "how-to," of the treatments discussed. The bibliotherapy resources are selected publications on topics relevant to the DVD content that may be helpful to clients or laypersons.

References are made to homework assignments contained at www.wiley.com/go/anxietywb that demonstrate selected therapeutic interventions discussed in the DVD.

In Appendix A, the correct and incorrect answers to all chapter review test questions are explained.

As a training process, we recommend that the facilitator play the DVD chapter by chapter, starting with the first. Participants are asked to watch the DVD and follow it in their workbook.

At the conclusion of each chapter, the *Companion Workbook* and *Facilitator's Guide* each have a section entitled Chapter Review. This section asks questions covering the major points of the chapter. The *Facilitator's Guide* has brief summaries of the answers to these chapter review questions. We recommend reading each of these questions, asking participants to briefly discuss them, and then summarizing the major teaching points as provided in the *Facilitator Guide*.

Following the Chapter Review section is a brief section entitled Chapter Review Test Questions. It contains test-style questions that can be asked of participants or taken by them as a self-test. The *Facilitator's Guide* contains the answers to these questions, which can then be reviewed. Appendix A of the *Facilitator's Guide* and Appendix A of the *Companion Workbook* contain explanations of all correct and incorrect answer options, if needed.

Finally, the *Facilitator's Guide* chapters each contain a section entitled For Discussion, which offers a selected discussion topic as well as talking points to help facilitate the discussion. This section is designed to offer facilitators the option of exploring a key concept further should he or she desire.

Chapter Points

This DVD is electronically marked with chapter points that delineate the beginning of major sections throughout the program. You may skip to any one of these chapter points in the video by clicking on the forward arrow. The chapter points for this program are as follows:

➤ DSM Criteria for Social Anxiety Disorder
➤ Six Steps to a Treatment Plan
➤ Introduction to ESTs for Social Anxiety Disorder
➤ Integrating ESTs for Social Anxiety Disorder into Treatment Planning
➤ Calming and Coping Skills
➤ Cognitive Restructuring
➤ Situational Exposure
➤ Social Skills Training
➤ Other Common Approaches to Treatment
➤ Relapse Prevention

Series Rationale

Evidence-based practice (EBP) is steadily becoming the standard of mental health-care as it has in medical healthcare. Borrowing from the Institute of Medicine's definition (Institute of Medicine, 2001), the American Psychological Association (APA) has defined EBP as "the integration of the best available research with clinical expertise in the context of patient characteristics, culture, and preferences" (American Psychological Association Presidential Task Force on Evidence-Based Practice [APA], 2006).

Professional organizations such as the American Psychological Association, the National Association of Social Workers, and the American Psychiatric Association, as well as consumer organizations such the National Alliance for the Mentally Ill (NAMI), are endorsing EBP. At the federal level, a major joint initiative of the National Institute of Mental Health and Department of Health and Human Services' Substance Abuse and Mental Health Services Administration (SAMHSA) focuses on promoting, implementing, and evaluating evidence-based mental health programs and practices within state mental health systems (APA, 2006). In some practice settings, EBP is even becoming mandated. It is clear that the call for evidence-based practice is being increasingly sounded.

Unfortunately, many mental healthcare providers cannot or do not stay abreast of results from clinical research and how these results can inform their practices. Although it has rightfully been argued that the relevance of some research to the clinician's needs is weak, there are products of clinical research whose efficacy has been well established and whose effectiveness in the community setting has received support. Clinicians and clinicians-in-training interested in empirically informing their treatments could benefit from educational programs that make this goal more easily attainable.

This series of DVDs and companion workbooks is designed to introduce clinicians and students to the process of empirically informing their psychotherapy treatment plans. The series begins with an introduction to the efforts to identify research-supported treatments and how the products of these efforts can be used to inform treatment planning. The other programs in the series focus on empirically informed treatment planning for each of several commonly seen clinical problems. In each problem-focused DVD, issues involved in defining or diagnosing the presenting problem are reviewed. Research-supported treatments for the problem are described, as well as the process used to identify them. Viewers are then systematically guided through the process of creating a treatment plan, and shown how the plan can be informed by goals, objectives, and interventions consistent with those of the identified research-supported treatments. Example vignettes of selected interventions are also provided.

This series is intended to be educational and informative in nature and not meant to be a substitute for clinical training in the specific interventions discussed and demonstrated. References to empirical support of the treatments described, clinical resource material, and training opportunities are provided.

Presenters

Figure I.1 Dr. Tim Bruce and Dr. Art Jongsma

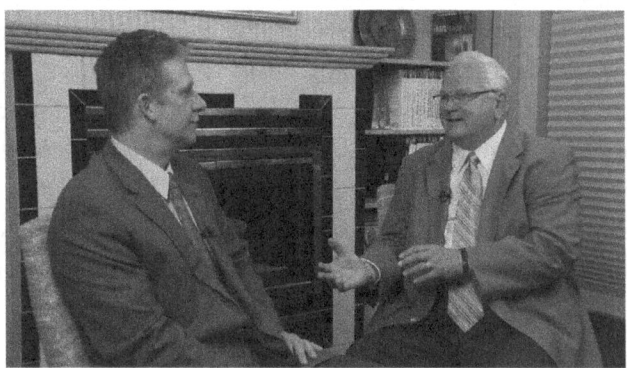

Dr. Art Jongsma is the Series Editor and coauthor of the Practice*Planners*® series[1] published by John Wiley & Sons. He has authored or coauthored more than 40 books in this series. Among the books included in this series are the highly regarded *The Complete Adult Psychotherapy Treatment Planner, The Adolescent* and *The Child Psychotherapy Treatment Planners*, and *The Addiction Treatment Planner*. All of these books along with *The Severe and Persistent Mental Illness Treatment Planner, The Family Therapy Treatment Planner, The Couples Psychotherapy Treatment Planner*, and *The Veterans and Active Duty Military Psychotherapy Treatment Planner* are informed with objectives and interventions that are supported by research evidence.

Dr. Jongsma also created the clinical record management software tool, Thera*Scribe*®, which uses point-and-click technology to easily develop, store, and print treatment plans, progress notes, and homework assignments. He has conducted treatment planning and software training workshops for mental health professionals around the world.

Dr. Jongsma's clinical career began as a psychologist in a large private psychiatric hospital. He worked in the hospital for about 10 years and then transitioned to outpatient work in his own private practice clinic, Psychological Consultants, in Grand Rapids, Michigan for 25 years. He has been writing best-selling books and software for mental health professionals since 1995.

---

[1]These books are updated frequently, check with the publisher for the latest editions.

Dr. Timothy Bruce is a Professor and Associate Chair of the Department of Psychiatry and Behavioral Medicine at the University of Illinois, College of Medicine in Peoria, Illinois, where he also directs medical student education. He is a licensed clinical psychologist who completed his graduate training at SUNY-Albany under the mentorship of Dr. David Barlow and his residency training at Wilford Hall Medical Center under the direction of Dr. Robert Klepac. In addition to maintaining an active clinical practice at the university, Dr. Bruce has authored numerous publications including books, professional journal articles, book chapters, and professional educational materials, many on the topic of evidence-based practice. Most recently, he has served as the contributing editor empirically informing Dr. Jongsma's best-selling Practice*Planners*® Series.

Dr. Bruce is also Executive Director of the Center for the Dissemination of Evidence-based Mental Health Practices, a state- and federally funded initiative to disseminate evidence-based psychological and pharmacological practices across Illinois. Highly recognized as an educator, Dr. Bruce has received nearly two dozen awards for his teaching of students and professionals during his career.

References

American Psychological Association Presidential Task Force on Evidence-Based Practice. (2006). Evidence-based practice in psychology. *American Psychologist, 61(4)*, 271–285.

Berghuis, D., Jongsma, A., and Bruce, T. (2006). *The severe and persistent mental illness treatment planner* (2nd ed.). Hoboken, NJ: John Wiley & Sons.

Dattilio, F., Jongsma, A., and Davis, S. (2009). *The family therapy treatment planner* (2nd ed.). Hoboken, NJ: John Wiley & Sons.

Institute of Medicine. (2001). *Crossing the quality chasm: A new health system for the 21st century*. Washington, DC: National Academy Press.

Jongsma, A., Peterson, M., & Bruce, T. (2006). *The complete adult psychotherapy treatment planner* (4th ed.). Hoboken, NJ: John Wiley & Sons.

Jongsma, A., Peterson, M., McInnis, W., & Bruce, T. (2006a). *The adolescent psychotherapy treatment planner* (4th ed.). Hoboken, NJ: John Wiley & Sons.

Jongsma, A., Peterson, M., McInnis, W., & Bruce, T. (2006b). *The child psychotherapy treatment planner* (4th ed.). Hoboken, NJ: John Wiley & Sons.

Moore, B., & Jongsma, A. (2009). *The veterans and active duty military psychotherapy treatment planner*. Hoboken, NJ: John Wiley & Sons.

Perkinson, R., Jongsma, A., & Bruce, T. (2009). *The addiction treatment planner* (4th ed.). Hoboken, NJ: John Wiley & Sons.

CHAPTER 1

What Are the DSM Criteria for Social Anxiety Disorder?

Chapter Review

1. What are the diagnostic criteria for social anxiety disorder (SAD)?

SOCIAL ANXIETY DISORDER

- Persistent fear of one or more social situations
- Fear that he/she will be humiliated, embarrassed, or otherwise evaluated negatively
- Anxiety or panic in response to the social situation
- Avoidance or endurance with distress
- Significant interference with the person's normal routine; occupational or academic functioning; social activities; or relationships; or there is marked distress about having the social anxiety

---

2. Name and discuss examples of commonly feared social performance and interactions.

- Some individuals with SAD show fear to only one or a few social situations, typically performance-type situations such as public speaking. Others show a more generalized fear of several situations, including both social performance and social interactions.

EXAMPLES OF COMMONLY FEARED PERFORMANCE SITUATIONS

- Speaking in public
- Formal (large groups) speaking?
- Informal (small groups) speaking?
- Writing in front of others
- Eating in front of others

(*continues*)

- Playing an instrument
- Playing sports
- Entering a room full of people
- Using a public toilet

EXAMPLES OF COMMONLY FEARED SOCIAL INTERACTIONS
- Socializing
- Going to a party
- Making "small talk"
- Eating lunch with peers
- Dating
- Asking a teacher for help
- Speaking to a boss at work
- Asking a salesclerk for help
- Asking for directions

Chapter Review Test Questions

1. What feature of SAD helps differentiate it from normal shyness?

   A. SAD may involve anxiety symptoms; shyness typically does not.

   B. SAD may involve public speaking fears; shyness typically does not.

   C. SAD involves clinically significant distress or disability; shyness typically does not.

   D. SAD and shyness are two names for the same thing.

   Answer: C

2. Which of the following is most likely to be feared and avoided by someone with SAD?

   A. An interactive classroom

   B. Driving an automobile

   C. Flying in a plane

   D. Listening to a public speaker

   Answer: A

Talking Points

Clients with social anxiety can show various behavioral presentations despite having the same fundamental fear. To facilitate a discussion of this issue, consider posing the following question: "How might clients with SAD show different manifestations of this same fundamental fear?

- This discussion may be facilitated by inviting participants to discuss previous or current clients, what they feared and avoided, and how this fear and avoidance still reflects the fundamental social nature of the fear (i.e., embarrassment, humiliation, rejection, negative evaluation by others).
- To facilitate this discussion, consider these questions:
  - Let's talk briefly about clients we've had with this diagnosis. What kinds of things did they fear doing or would avoid?
  - What was it they feared could happen?
  - What are the common themes emerging in their fear and avoidance?

Chapter Reference

American Psychiatric Association. (2000). *Diagnostic and statistical manual of mental disorders.* (4th ed., text revised). Washington, DC: American Psychiatric Association.

2

What Are the Six Steps in Building a Treatment Plan?

Chapter Review

1. What are the six steps involved in developing a psychotherapy treatment plan?

> Step 1: Identify primary and secondary problems
>
> Step 2: Describe the problem's behavioral manifestations (symptom pattern)
>
> Step 3: Make a diagnosis based on DSM/ICD criteria
>
> Step 4: Specify long-term goals
>
> Step 5: Create short-term objectives
>
> Step 6: Select therapeutic interventions

Chapter Review Test Questions

1. A psychotherapy treatment plan can be drawn up without a diagnosis. For example, a good case formulation can be the basis of therapy. Why is it important to consider the diagnosis when developing a plan that could be informed by empirically supported treatments (ESTs)?

    A. A diagnosis is necessary to judge response to the EST.

    B. It is not necessary to consider diagnosis in empirically informed treatment planning.

    C. Some ESTs were developed and studied using diagnosis as inclusion criteria.

    D. Treatment may require medication, which typically requires diagnosis to be specified.

    Answer: C

2. The statement, "Identify, challenge, and change biased self-talk supportive of social anxiety" is an example of which of the following steps in a treatment plan?

   A. A primary problem
   B. A short-term objective
   C. A symptom manifestation
   D. A treatment intervention
   Answer: B

Talking Point

What is the relationship between short-term objectives (STOs) and treatment interventions (TIs) in a treatment plan?

- In essence, STOs are desired actions of the client, while TIs are the therapist's actions designed to help clients achieve the objectives.

Chapter References

American Psychological Association Presidential Task Force on Evidence-Based Practice. (2006). Evidence-based practice in psychology. *American Psychologist, 61* (4), 271–285.

Jongsma, A. (2005). Psychotherapy treatment plan writing. In G. P. Koocher, J. C. Norcross, & S. S. Hill (Eds.), *Psychologists' desk reference* (2nd ed., pp. 232–236). New York: Oxford University Press.

Jongsma, A. Peterson, M., & Bruce, T. (2006). *The complete adult psychotherapy treatment planner* (4th ed.). Hoboken, NJ: John Wiley & Sons.

3

What Is the Brief History of the Empirically Supported Treatments Movement?

Chapter Review

1. How did Division 12 of the APA identify empirically supported treatments (ESTs)?

> • This group evaluated psychotherapy outcome literature using two primary sets of criteria for judging the evidence base supporting any particular therapy. One was termed *well-established*, the other *probably efficacious*.

2. What are the primary differences between *well-established* and *probably efficacious* criteria used to identify treatments?

> • The criteria for well-established treatment required at least two randomized, placebo-controlled trials (RCTs) or two randomized trials comparing the treatment to an already established treatment, or a large series of single case design studies. In these studies, treatment manuals had to be used, and characteristics of the client sample had to be specified. Finally, replication by different investigators had to have been demonstrated.
>
> • The criteria for probably efficacious treatment could be met with two demonstrations of efficacy over a wait-list control. This is a lower level of evidence than for the well-established treatment: It rules out only that the condition being treated does not remit on its own.
>
> • Alternatively, one or more RCTs or randomized trials comparing the treatment to an already established treatment in which manuals were used, client characteristics were specified, but independent replication had *not* been demonstrated would suffice.
>
> • As with well-established criteria, a single case series, but of smaller size than required in well-established, could be used.
>
> ———
> See Figure 3.1 for use if more detailed questions arise.

─────────────────── **Figure 3.1** ───────────────────

Specific Criteria for Well-Established and Probably Efficacious Treatments

Criteria For Well-Established Treatments

For a psychological treatment to be considered *well-established*, the evidence base supporting it had to be characterized by the following:

I. At least two good between group design experiments demonstrating efficacy in one or more of the following ways:

    A. Superior (statistically significantly so) to pill or psychological placebo or to another treatment

    B. Equivalent to an already established treatment in experiments with adequate sample sizes

OR

II. A large series of single case design experiments (n > 9) demonstrating efficacy; these experiments must:

    A. Use good experimental designs

    B. Compare the intervention to another treatment, as in IA

Further Criteria For Both I And II

III. Experiments must be conducted with treatment manuals.

IV. Characteristics of the client samples must be clearly specified.

V. Effects must have been demonstrated by at least two different investigators or investigating teams.

Criteria For Probably Efficacious Treatments

For a psychological treatment to be considered *probably efficacious*, the evidence base supporting it had to meet the following criteria:

I. Two experiments showing the treatment is superior (statistically significantly so) to a waiting-list control group

OR

II. One or more experiments meeting the well-established treatment criteria IA or IB, III, and IV, but not V

OR

III. A small series of single case design experiments (n > 3) otherwise meeting well-established treatment criteria

─────────────────

Adapted from: Chambless, D. L., Baker, M. J., Baucom, D. H., Beutler, L. E., Calhoun, K. S., Crits-Christoph, P., Daiuto, A., DeRubeis, R., Detweiler, J., Haaga, D. A. F., Bennett Johnson, S., McCurry, S., Mueser, K. T., Pope, K. S., Sanderson, W. C., Shoham, V., Stickle, T., Williams, D. A., & Woody, S. R. (1998). Update on empirically validated therapies, II. *The Clinical Psychologist, 51(1)*, 3–16.

3. Where can information about ESTs and evidence-based practices be found?

- In 1999, The Society of Clinical Psychology, Division 12, took full ownership of maintaining the growing list. The current list and information center can be found on its Web site, at www.psychologicaltreatments.org.

- Great Britain was at the forefront of the effort to identify evidence-based treatments and develop guidelines for practice. The latest products of their work can be found at the Web site for the National Institute for Health and Clinical Excellence (NICE): www.nice.org.uk.

- The Substance Abuse and Mental Health Service Administration (SAMHSA) has also begun an initiative to evaluate, identify, and provide information on various mental health practices. Their work, entitled, "The National Registry of Evidence-based Programs and Practices," can be found online at www.nrepp.samhsa.gov.

- The Web site www.therapyadvisor.com provides descriptions, references to empirical support, clinical training materials, and training opportunities for many of the empirically supported treatment identified by the original Division 12 review groups.

Chapter Review Test Questions

1. Which statement best describes the process used to identify ESTs?

    A. Consumers of mental health services nominated therapies.

    B. Experts came to a consensus based on their experiences with the treatments.

    C. Researchers submitted their works.

    D. Task groups reviewed the literature using clearly defined selection criteria for ESTs.

    Answer: D

2. Based on the differences in their criteria, in which of the following ways are *well-established* treatments different than those classified as *probably efficacious*?

    A. Only probably efficacious treatments allowed the use of single case design experiments.

    B. Only well-established treatments allowed studies comparing the treatment to a psychological placebo.

    C. Only well-established treatments required demonstration by at least two different, independent investigators or investigating teams.

    D. Only well-established treatments allowed studies comparing the treatment to a pill placebo.

    Answer: C

Talking Point

Why would it be important to have treatment results replicated by independent investigators investigative teams?

- Discuss factors in some studies that can lead to *allegiance effects*, in which the positive outcome is found only by investigators who are, generally speaking, advocates of the therapy. Examples could include demand characteristics, advanced training in the techniques, and biased assessment of treatment response.

Chapter References

Chambless, D. L., & Ollendick, T. H. (2001). Empirically supported psychological interventions: Controversies and evidence. *Annual Review of Psychology, 52,* 685–716.

Chambless, D. L., Sanderson, W. C., Shoham, V., Bennett Johnson, S., Pope, K. S., Crits-Christoph, P., et al. (1996). An update on empirically validated therapies. *The Clinical Psychologist, 49,* 5–18.

Chambless, D. L., Baker, M. J., Baucom, D. H., Beutler, L. E., Calhoun, K. S., Crits-Christoph, P., et al. (1998). Update on empirically validated therapies, II.*The Clinical Psychologist, 51(1),* 3–16.

Gatz, M., Fiske, A., Fox, L. S., Kaskie, B., Kasl-Godley, J. E., et al. (1998). Empirically validated psychological treatments for older adults. *Journal of Mental Health and Aging, 41,* 9–46.

Kendall, P. C., & Chambless, D. L. (Eds.). (1998). Empirically supported psychological therapies [Special issue]. *Journal of Consulting and Clinical Psychology, 66* (3)151–167.

Lonigan, C. J., & Elbert, J. C. (Eds.). (1998). Special issue on empirically supported psychosocial interventions for children. *Journal of Clinical Child Psychology, 27,* 138–226.

Nathan, P. E., & Gorman, J. M. (Eds.). (1998). *A guide to treatments that work.* New York: Oxford University Press.

Nathan, P. E., & Gorman, J. M. (Eds.). (2002*). A guide to treatments that work* (2nd ed.). New York: Oxford University Press.

Nathan, P. E., & Gorman, J. M. (Eds.). (2007). *A guide to treatments that work* (3rd ed.). New York: Oxford University Press.

Spirito, A. (Ed.). (1999). Empirically supported treatments in pediatric psychology [Special issue]. *Journal of Pediatric Psychology, 24,* 87–174.

4

What Are the Identified Empirically Supported Treatments for Social Anxiety Disorder?

Chapter Review

1. What therapies have been identified as having well-established efficacy in the treatment of social anxiety disorder (SAD)?

- Cognitive and behavioral treatments have met the criteria for a well-established EST (see Teachman at www.psychologicaltreatments.org).
- Cognitive and behavioral therapies for SAD refer to a variety of techniques, including cognitive restructuring, exposure, and skills training. In addition, skills used for managing anxiety may be trained. There is also a strong ongoing emphasis on psychoeducation.

---

2. What are the primary interventions used in these therapies?

Well-established ESTs for Social Anxiety Disorder

COGNITIVE AND BEHAVIORAL THERAPIES TYPICALLY INCLUDE
- Cognitive restructuring
- Exposure
- Social skills training (if needed)

MAY OR MAY NOT INCLUDE
- Anxiety management skills training
- Psychoeducation

Chapter Review Test Questions

1. Which statement best characterizes the use of social skills training in CBT for SAD?

    A. It is a key feature of treatment for SAD and always trained.

    B. It is not a key feature of treatment for SAD and is not trained.

    C. It is trained depending upon an assessment of skill deficits.

D. It is trained only if public speaking fears are evident.

Answer: C

2. In the treatment of SAD, the practice of asking the client to repeatedly engage in feared and/or avoided social activities is called:

A. Applied relaxation
B. Cognitive restructuring
C. Exposure
D. Psychoeducation

Answer: C

Talking Points

Traditional behavioral therapies for social anxiety prescribed exposure to what clients fear and avoid, but cognitive therapy also involves engaging in activities that are feared and avoided. What is the difference between these two seemingly similar prescriptions?

- As mentioned in the DVD, exposure derived from early behavioral therapies, like systematic desensitization, and was originally based on conditioning theories— including two-factor theory, counter-conditioning, and classical extinction. Those models guided how the procedure was conducted, and helps explain why it evolved from systematic desensitization to today's versions.

- From the cognitive therapy perspective, however, the same action (exposure) was seen as an arena for conducting the behavioral experiments used in this therapy. Behavioral experiments are therapeutic exercises in which the client's fearful thoughts are turned into predictions, alternatives to them are generated, and then both are tested in these real-life "experiments." In anxiety disorders, this commonly involves testing fearful predictions by engaging in a feared social performance or interaction.

- Behavioral, cognitive, and cognitive behavioral therapists may differ in their particular conceptualization of the mechanism(s) through which exposure achieves the efficacy it has demonstrated.

Chapter References

Empirical Support

Cognitive Behavioral Therapy

Butler, A. C., Chapman, J. E., Forman, E. M., & Beck, A. T. (2006). The empirical status of cognitive-behavioral therapy: A review of meta-analyses. *Clinical Psychology Review, 26,* 17–31.

Cottraux, J., Note, I., Albuisson, E., Yao, S. N., Note, B., Mollard, E., et al. (2000). Cognitive behavior therapy versus supportive therapy in social phobia: A randomized controlled trial. *Psychotherapy and Psychosomatics, 69,* 137–46.

Davidson, J. R. T., Foa, E. B., Huppert, J. D., Keefe, F., Franklin, M., Compton, J., et al. (2004). Fluoxetine, comprehensive cognitive behavioral therapy, and placebo in generalized social phobia. *Archives of General Psychiatry, 61,* 1005–1013.

Gelernter, C. S., Uhde, T. W., Cimbolic, P., Arnkoff, D. B., Vittone, B. J., Tancer, M. E., & Bartko, J. J. (1991). Cognitive-behavioral and pharmacological treatments of social phobia. *Archives of General Psychiatry, 48,* 938–945.

Gould, R. A., Buckminster, S., Pollack, M. H., Otto, M. W., & Yap, L. (1997). Cognitive-behavioral and pharmacological treatment for social phobia: A meta-analysis. *Clinical Psychology: Science and Practice, 4,* 291–306.

Heimberg, R. G., Dodge, C. S., Hope, D. A., Kennedy, C. R., Zollo, L. J., & Becker, R. E. (2000). Cognitive behavioral group treatment for social phobia: Comparison with a credible placebo control. *Cognitive Therapy and Research, 14,* 1–23.

Heimberg, R. G., Liebowitz, M. R., Hope, D. A., Schneier, F. R., Holt, C. S., Welkowitz, L. A., et al. (1998). Cognitive behavioral group therapy versus phenelzine therapy for social phobia. *Archives of General Psychiatry, 55,* 1133–1141.

Heimberg, R. G., Salzman, D., Holt, C. S., & Blendell, K. (1993). Cognitive behavioral group treatment of social phobia: *Effectiveness at 5-year follow-up. Cognitive Therapy and Research, 17,* 325–339.

Hofmann, S. G. (2004). Cognitive mediation of treatment change in social phobia. *Journal of Consulting and Clinical Psychology, 72,* 392–399.

McNally, R., Bryant, R.A., & Ehlers, A. (2003). Does early psychological intervention promote recovery from posttraumatic stress? *Psychological Science in the Public Interest, 4,* 45–79.

Otto, M. W., Pollack, M. H., Gould, R. A., Worthington, J. J., McArdle, E. T., Rosenbaum, J. F., et al. (2000). A comparison of the efficacy of clonazepam and cognitive-behavioral group therapy for the treatment of social phobia. *Journal of Anxiety Disorders, 14,* 345–58.

Cognitive Therapy

Clark, D. M., Ehlers, A., McManus, F., Hackmati, A., Fennell, M., Campbell, H., et al. (2003). Cognitive therapy versus fluoxetine in generalized social phobia: A randomized placebo-controlled trial. *Journal of Consulting and Clinical Psychology, 71,* 1058–1067.

Stangier, U., Heidenreich, T., Peitz, M., Lauterbach, W., & Clark, D. M. (2003). Cognitive therapy for social phobia: Individual versus group treatment. *Behaviour Research and Therapy, 41,* 991–1007.

Taylor, S., Woody, S., Koch, W. J., McLean, P., Paterson, R. J., & Anderson, K. W. (1997). Cognitive restructuring in the treatment of social phobia: Efficacy and mode of action. *Behavior Modification, 21,* 487–511.

Exposure Therapy

Hope, D. A., Heimberg, R. G., & Bruch, M. A. (1995). Dismantling cognitive-behavioral group therapy for social phobia. *Behaviour Research and Therapy, 33,* 637–650.

Salaberria, K., & Echeburua, E. (1998). Long-term outcome of cognitive therapy's contribution to self-exposure in vivo to the treatment of generalized social phobia. *Behavior Modification, 22,* 262–84.

Scholing, A., & Emmelkamp, P. M. G. (1996). Treatment of generalized social phobia: Results at long-term follow-up. *Behaviour Research and Therapy, 34,* 447–452.

Turner, S. M., Beidel, D. C., & Jacob, R. G. (1994). Social phobia: A comparison of behavior therapy and atenolol. *Journal of Consulting and Clinical Psychology, 62,* 350–358.

Social Skills Training

Herbert, J. D., Gaudiano, B. A., Rheingold, A. A., Myers, V. H., Dalrymple, K. L., & Nolan, B. M. (2005). Social skills training augments the effectiveness of cognitive behavior group therapy for social anxiety disorder. *Behavior Therapy, 36,* 125–138.

Mersch, P. P. A., Emmelkamp, P. M. G., Bögels, S. M., & van der Sleen, J. (1989). Social phobia: Individual response patterns and the effects of behavioral and cognitive interventions. *Behaviour Research and Therapy, 27,* 421–434.

Wlazlo, Z., Schroeder-Harting, K., Hand, I., Kaiser, G., & Münchau, N. (1990). Exposure in vivo versus social skills training for social phobia: Long-term outcome and differential effects. *Behaviour Research and Therapy, 28,* 181–193.

Relaxation Training

Jerremalm, A., Jansson, L., & Öst, L.-G. (1986). Cognitive and physiological reactivity and the effects of different behavioral methods in the treatment of social phobia. *Behaviour Research and Therapy, 24,* 171–180.

Olsson-Jerremalm, A. (1988). Applied relaxation in the treatment of phobias. *Scandinavian Journal of Behaviour Therapy, 17,* 97–110.

Öst, L.-G., Jerremalm, A., & Johansson, J. (1981). Individual response patterns and the effects of different behavioral methods in the treatment of social phobia. *Behaviour Research and Therapy, 19,* 1–16.

Systematic Desensitization

Lent, R. W., Russell, R. K., & Zamostny, K. P. (1981). Comparison of cue-controlled desensitization, rational restructuring, and a credible placebo in the treatment of speech anxiety. *Journal of Consulting and Clinical Psychology, 49,* 608–610.

Paul, G. L. (1967). Insight versus desensitization in psychotherapy two years after termination. *Journal of Consulting Psychology, 31*, 333–348.

Paul, G. L., & Shannon, D. T. (1966). Treatment of anxiety through systematic desensitization in therapy groups. *Journal of Abnormal Psychology, 71*, 123–135.

Teachman, B. A. *Social phobia and public speaking anxiety.* **Retrieved September 3, 2009 from www.psychologicaltreatments.org.**

Clinical Resources

Antony, M. M., & Rowa, K. (2008). *Social phobia.* Göttingen, Germany: Hogrefe and Huber Publishers,

Antony, M. M., & Swinson, R. P. (2000). *The shyness and social anxiety workbook: Proven, step-by-step techniques for overcoming your fear.* Oakland, CA: New Harbinger Publications.

Benson, H. (1975, 2000). *The relaxation response.* New York: Avon. (Note: Benson conducted numerous studies of the benefits of relaxation and various medical applications.)

Bernstein, D. A., Borkovec, T. D., & Hazlett-Stevens, H. (2000). *New directions in progressive muscle relaxation: A guidebook for helping professionals.* Westbury, CT: Praeger Publishers.

Hope, D. A., Heimberg, R. G. , & Turk, C. L. (2006). Therapist guide for *Managing social anxiety: A cognitive-behavioral therapy approach.* New York: Oxford University Press.

Heimberg , R. G., & Becker, R. E. (2002). *Cognitive-behavioral group therapy for social phobia: Basic mechanisms and clinical strategies.* New York: Guilford Press.

Jacobson, E. (1938). *Progressive relaxation.* Chicago: University of Chicago Press.

Liberman, R. P., King, L. W., De Risi, W. J., & McCann, M. (1975). *Personal effectiveness: Guiding people to assert themselves and improve their social skills.* Champaign, IL: Research Press.

Markaway, B., Carmin, C., Pollard, C., & Flynn, T. (1992). *Dying of embarrassment: Help for social anxiety and phobia.* Oakland, CA: New Harbinger Publications.

Ost, L. G. (1987). Applied relaxation: Description of a coping technique and review of controlled studies. *Behaviour Research and Therapy, 25*, 397–409.

Kase, L., & Monarth, H. (2007). *The confident speaker.* New York: McGraw-Hill.

Rapee, R. M. (1998). *Overcoming shyness and social phobia: A step-by-step guide.* Northvale, NJ: Jason Aronson.

Trower, P., Bryant, B. M., & Argyle, M. (1978), *Social skills and mental health.* London, UK: Methuen.

Turk, C. L., Heimberg, R. C., & Hope, D. A. (2007). Social anxiety disorder. In D. H. Barlow (Ed.), *Clinical handbook of psychological disorders* (4th ed.). New York: Guilford Press.

Bibliotherapy Resources

Alberti, R. E., & Emmons, M. L. (2001). *Your perfect right: Assertiveness and equality in your life and relationships* (8th ed.). Atascadero, CA: Impact Publishers.

Antony, M. M., & Swinson, R. P. (2000). *The shyness and social anxiety workbook: Proven, step-by-step techniques for overcoming your fear.* Oakland, CA: New Harbinger Publications.

Butler, G. (1999). *Overcoming social anxiety and shyness: A self-help guide using cognitive behavioral techniques.* London, UK: Robinson.

Garner, A. (1997). *Conversationally speaking: Tested new ways to increase your personal and social effectiveness.* Los Angeles: Lowell House.

Markway, B.G., Carmin, C.N., Pollard, C.A., & Flynn, T. (1992). *Dying of embarrassment: Help for social anxiety and phobia.* Oakland, CA: New Harbinger Publications.

Rapee, R. M. (1998). *Overcoming shyness and social phobia: A step-by-step guide.* Northvale, NJ: Jason Aronson.

Schneier, F., & Welkowitz, L. (1996). *The hidden face of shyness: Understanding and overcoming social anxiety.* New York: Avon Books.

Soifer, S., Zgourides, G.D., Himle, J., & Pickering, N.L. (2001). *Shy bladder syndrome: Your step-by-step guide to overcoming paruresis.* Oakland, CA: New Harbinger Publications.

Stein, M. B., & Walker, J. R. (2001). *Triumph over shyness: Conquering shyness and social anxiety.* New York: McGraw Hill.

CHAPTER 5

How Do You Integrate Empirically Supported Treatments into Treatment Planning?

This section of the DVD takes the viewer through each step in the process of integrating Empirically Supported Treatments (ESTs) into a treatment plan. It discusses each step of treatment planning for the identified problem (i.e., behavioral definitions, goals, objectives, and treatment interventions) and provides examples of how each can be written, with the objectives and interventions reflecting content consistent with indicated ESTs. In this *Guide*, we have reproduced the examples shown on the DVD and included in the *Companion Workbook*. This gives you the option of stopping the DVD to discuss an example, or simply letting it play.

In the section on objectives and interventions shown on the DVD, vignettes are shown that demonstrate an aspect of selected interventions. Each vignette is followed by a brief critique of the demonstration. The script of these vignettes, comments made in the critique, and a section allowing viewers to further critique are included in this *Guide* as well as the *Companion Workbook*. You can elect to facilitate this additional critique by viewers, or not.

Following selected vignettes, references may be made to homework assignments that may be found and reprinted at www.wiley.com/go/anxietywb. These assignments demonstrate selected therapeutic interventions consistent with those discussed in the DVD. These can be reviewed and discussed at the facilitator's discretion.

As in previous chapters, each vignette is followed by review questions, test questions, and an optional discussion question for use by the facilitator.

Integrating ESTs into Treatment Planning

Construction of an empirically informed treatment plan for social anxiety disorder (SAD) involves integrating objectives and treatment interventions consistent with identified ESTs into a client's treatment plan after you have determined that the client's primary problem fits those described in the target population of the EST research.

Of course, implementing ESTs must be done in consideration of important client, therapist, and therapeutic relationship factors, consistent with the definition of evidence-based practice.

Definitions

The behavioral definition statements describe *how the problem manifests itself in the client*. Your assessment will need to identify which features best characterize your client's presentation.

When the primary problem reflects a recognized psychiatric diagnosis, the behavioral definition statements are usually closely aligned with diagnostic criteria such as those provided in the DSM or ICD.

Examples of common SAD definition statements are the following:

➤ Expresses excessive, unrealistic fear and worry about social performance or interactions
➤ Admits to constant worry about social interaction
➤ Tends to feel blamed by others for the slightest imperfection or mistake
➤ Reports symptoms of autonomic hyperactivity in social situations (e.g., cardiac palpitations, shortness of breath, sweaty palms, dry mouth, trouble swallowing, nausea, diarrhea) in response to social situations
➤ Demonstrates symptoms of muscle tension
➤ Reports symptoms of hypervigilance in social settings (e.g., feeling constantly on edge, difficulty concentrating, sleep problems, irritability)
➤ Escapes or avoids situations that require a degree of interpersonal contact
➤ Reluctant involvement in social situations out of fear of saying or doing something foolish or of becoming emotional in front of others
➤ Debilitating performance anxiety and/or avoidance of required social performance demands
➤ Lacks the necessary social skills to initiate and maintain relationships
➤ Alienates self from others due to socially inappropriate behavior
➤ Others

Goals

Goals are broad statements describing what you and the client would like the result of therapy to be. One statement may suffice but more than one can be used in the treatment plan.

Examples of common goal statements for SAD are the following:

➤ Interact socially without undue fear or anxiety

> ➤ Perform socially without undue fear or debilitating anxiety
> ➤ Develop the essential social skills necessary to function in social situations without undue anxiety
> ➤ Develop the ability to form relationships
> ➤ Reach a personal balance between solitary time and interpersonal interaction with others
> ➤ Form social relationships that enhance the quality of life
> ➤ Others

Objectives and Interventions

Objectives are statements that describe *small, observable steps the client must achieve* toward attaining the goal of successful treatment. Intervention statements describe the *actions taken by the therapist* to assist the client in achieving his/her objectives. Each objective must be paired with at least one intervention.

Assessment

All approaches to quality treatment start with a thorough assessment of the nature and history of the client's presenting problems. EST approaches to treatment rely on a thorough psychosocial assessment of the nature, history, and severity of the problem as experienced by the client. Table 5.1 contains examples of assessment objectives and interventions.

Table 5.1   Assessment Objectives and Interventions

Objectives	Interventions
1. Describe the history and nature of social fears and avoidance.	1. Focus on developing a level of trust with the client; provide support and empathy to encourage the client to feel safe in expressing his/her social anxiety. 2. Assess the client's history of social fears and avoidance to date, including the frequency, intensity, and duration of representative symptoms. 3. Assess the nature of any stimulus, thoughts, or situations that precipitate the client's social fear and/or avoidance.
2. Keep a daily journal of social situations that cause anxious thoughts, feelings, and avoidant actions.	1. Assign the client to keep a daily record of social anxiety, including a description of each situation that caused anxious feelings, the rating of anxiety, using subjective units of distress (SUDs), and thoughts that triggered the anxiety; process the journal material and help the client uncover the dysfunctional, distorted thoughts that fueled the social anxiety.
3. Complete psychological testing or objective questionnaires for assessing social anxiety and social skills.	1. Administer to the client tests designed to assess social anxiety and social skills (e.g., Social Phobia and Anxiety Inventory [SPAI], the Social Interaction Anxiety Scale [SIAS], the Social Phobia Scale [SPS], Social Reticence Scale [SRS], or the Social Skills Inventory [SSI]); score and give feedback to the client; re-administer as needed to assess outcome.

Table 5.2   Psychoeducational Objectives and Interventions

Objectives	Interventions
4. Verbalize an accurate understanding of the vicious cycle of social anxiety and avoidance.	1. Discuss how social anxiety derives from cognitive biases that over-estimate the likelihood and manageability of negative evaluation by others; undervalue one's self-efficacy; distress; and often lead to unnecessary avoidance that maintains the fear. 2. Assign the client to read psychoeducational chapters of books or treatment manuals on social anxiety that explain the cycle of social anxiety and avoidance.
5. Verbalize an understanding of the rationale for treatment of social anxiety.	1. Discuss how cognitive restructuring and exposure serve as an arena to desensitize learned fear, build social skills and confidence, and reality-test biased thoughts. 2. Assign the client to read about cognitive restructuring and exposure-based therapy in chapters of books or treatment manuals on social anxiety (e.g., *Managing Social Anxiety* by Hope, Heimberg, Juster, & Turk; *Dying of Embarrassment* by Markaway, Carmin, Pollard, & Flynn).

Psychoeducation

A typical feature of many ESTs for social anxiety disorder is initial and ongoing psychoeducation. A common emphasis is helping the client learn about social anxiety, the treatment, and its rationale. Often, *books or other reading material are recommended to the client* to supplement psychoeducation done in session. It is important to instill hope in the client and have them on board as a partner in the treatment process. With ESTs, discussing their demonstrated efficacy with the client can facilitate this. Table 5.2 contains examples of psychoeducation objectives and interventions for social anxiety disorder.

Calming and Coping Skills

Although not all EST approaches to social anxiety use anxiety management techniques, there are those that do. Common skills include applied relaxation and cognitive coping strategies.

In applied relaxation, clients are taught how to achieve relaxation through progressive muscle relaxation (PMR). PMR is an exercise in which the client is taught how to systematically relax muscle groups, by tensing and releasing tension, until complete body relaxation is accomplished. As the client becomes more skilled in its use, the exercise is typically condensed so it can be applied rapidly in various life situations—something termed *rapid relaxation*. Once rapid relaxation is mastered, the client induces relaxation in the presence of social cues until anxiety associated with them is decreased.

When coping skills for managing social anxiety are trained, a common approach includes some combination of rapid relaxation, thought-stopping, and attentional refocusing. The purpose of thought-stopping (silently but assertively saying to oneself the word "stop") is to a halt train of thought that triggers anxious feelings. The purpose of attentional refocusing (changing from an anxious internal focus on anxiety and doubt to an external focus on the requirements of the social task) is to reduce anxiety generated by thinking about internal physiological sensations and critical self-talk.

These strategies are designed to facilitate social functioning by focusing attention on the requirements of the social task, while allowing anxiety to diminish. A summary of the calming and coping procedure follows:

1. Implement psychoeducation surrounding using coping skills to manage social anxiety.
2. Teach Jacobson's deep muscle relaxation method, including systematically tensing and relaxing sequential muscle groups.
3. Gradually reduce the number of muscle groups focused on until rapid relaxation can be induced within several seconds using trigger words like "be calm" or "relax."
4. Emphasize using evenly paced diaphragmatic breathing.
5. Teach the importance of shifting from internal focus of physiological changes to the demands and responsibilities of the external situation.
6. Teach the client to silently shout "stop!" to self to terminate thinking anxious thoughts and replace negative thoughts with positive thoughts.
7. Use role-play and behavioral rehearsal in session to apply the calming and coping skills to social anxiety cues.
8. Assign the use of rapid relaxation, paced breathing, and maintaining external focus as coping skills to be used in the face of social anxiety cues in daily living.
9. Review the use of calming and coping skills, reinforcing success and redirecting for failure.

Table 5.3 contains an objective and interventions that show how calming and coping skills can be described in the social anxiety disorder treatment plan.

Table 5.3   Calming and Coping Objective and Interventions

Objective	Interventions
6. Learn and implement calming and coping strategies to reduce overall anxiety and manage anxiety when heightened.	1. Teach the client relaxation, thought-stopping, and attentional focusing skills (e.g., staying focused externally and on behavioral goals; using muscular relaxation and evenly paced diaphragmatic breathing, as needed, to ride the wave of anxiety). 2. Assign the client to read about calming and coping strategies in books or treatment manuals on social anxiety.

Demonstration Vignette

Calming and Coping Skills

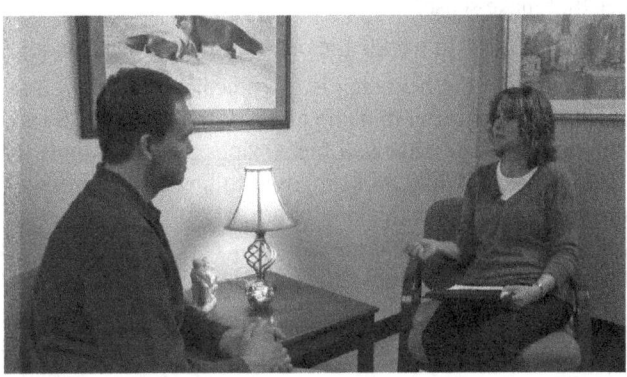

Here we present the transcript of the dialogue depicted in the calming and coping skills training vignette.

Therapist: Okay, in some of your previous sessions and in your homework you've practiced the muscle relaxation to calm yourself down. So how is that going?

Client: It's going pretty well, but I still have a lot of anxiety.

Therapist: Well, the relaxation is just part of managing your anxiety. It's focused on the physical side, and it's used to help maintain some level of calm. We want to keep doing that, but as we've discussed, a primary source of anxiety has to do with what your mind is focused on. For example, let's say you are relaxed and thinking about something calm, like lying on the beach.

Client: Pretty nice. Okay.

Therapist: Then, while relaxed, you suddenly start thinking about something bad happening to you, like you walk into a room full of people and they all start laughing, and you assume that they're laughing about you.

Client: Right, I see. Not so relaxed anymore.

Therapist: Right, and in social situations, your goal is to keep your focus off things that will make you anxious, like exactly what your heart is doing or what that guy who's laughing is thinking about, and you want to keep your mind on what you're going to do in that social situation. Does that make sense?

Client: Yep, perfect sense.

Therapist: So, let's talk about what you can do if your mind starts to wander off.

Client: Okay, sounds good.

Therapist: The first thing I'd like you to try is a simple technique called "thought-stopping."

Client: Thought-stopping? What's that?

Therapist: It helps you to take control and stop the focus on negative things ... like the thought "I'm going to make a fool of myself" or "People will laugh at me." You can usually tell when you

(continues)

are focused on negative thoughts by paying attention to how you feel. So whenever you start to have an anxious thought, I want you to shout the word STOP in your mind without making a sound. Sometimes it helps to even picture a big red stop sign in your head. Does that make sense?

Client: I think so. Shout "STOP" to myself the minute I start to have an anxious thought.

Therapist: That's right, and then the next step is to immediately bring yourself back to what you are supposed to be doing and thinking about at that moment. So you redirect your focus away from thoughts that make you feel anxious and focus on what is going on around you. You ask yourself, "What am I supposed to be doing right now?" Focus on the here and now. You want to stop thinking about what's making you anxious or your heart rate or your sweaty palms ... and instead think about what you want to say or do at the moment. Does that make sense?

Client: It does. [He nods]

Therapist: So let me show you how it works. Let's say I have to walk into a room full of people—some of them I know and some I don't know. Before I go in, I calm myself down using the rapid relaxation skills, like this—[breathe deep and exhale slowly]. Then a thought enters my mind that tells me I won't know what to say after I say hello. Immediately, I say "STOP" in my mind and picture a big red stop sign in my head. Then I refocus my attention and take my mind off the negative thought and think about what I would like to do in this situation. I think about why I am here and who do I know that I can talk to. I think about Jack, who is standing over there, and how I can ask him about his son's basketball game last night. So you see how this works?

Client: Yeah.

Therapist: I used relaxation, thought-stopping, and refocusing skills all together. Okay? Now you try it.

Critique of the Calming and Coping Skills Demonstration Vignette

The following points were made in the critique:

➤ The therapist is moving from somatic calming or relaxation to cognitive coping skills.

➤ Emphasis is on attentional refocusing on the external task and away from the negative self-talk or physiological symptoms of anxiety.

➤ The vignette nicely pairs relaxation with attentional refocusing and thought-stopping.

➤ Some therapists do not use explicit calming and coping skills, but rather simply encourage the client to focus on accomplishing the goals of the social task.

Additional points that could be made:

➤ When anticipatory social anxiety is a problem, thought-stopping can also be used, refocusing the mind on the likely successful outcome of an encounter or a pleasant, relaxing thought. This is usually done after the client has challenged the fearful predictions, developed the alternative, and then wants to minimize time spent revisiting the fearful prediction.

➤ Cognitive restructuring can be used in conjunction with these techniques to change biased messages that are triggering anxiety.

➤ It is not unusual to gradually shift from the explicit use of these skills to not using them as therapy progresses and client confidence increases.

Comments you would like to make:

_____

_____

_____

Homework: The homework exercise "Making Use of the Thought Stopping Technique" (see www.wiley.com/go/anxietywb) is an example of assigning the thought-stopping strategy as a stand-alone method.

Calming and Coping Skills Review

1. What are examples of calming and coping skills that may be trained for managing social anxiety?

CALMING AND COPING SKILLS FOR SOCIAL ANXIETY
- Rapid Relaxation
- Thought-Stopping
- Attentional Refocusing

---

2. How is the calming and coping skills procedure summarized?

SUMMARY OF THE CALMING AND COPING SKILLS PROCEDURE
1. Implement psychoeducation surrounding using coping skills to manage social anxiety.
2. Teach Jacobson's deep muscle relaxation method including systematically tensing and relaxing sequential muscle groups.
3. Gradually reduce the number of muscle groups focused on until rapid relaxation can be induced within several seconds using trigger words like "be calm" or "relax."
4. Emphasize using evenly paced diaphragmatic breathing.
5. Teach the importance of shifting from internal focus of physiological changes to the demands and responsibilities of the external situation.

(continues)

6. Teach the client to silently shout "stop!" to self to terminate thinking anxious thoughts and replace negative thoughts with positive thoughts.

7. Use role play and behavioral rehearsal in session to apply the calming and coping skills to social anxiety cues.

8. Assign the use of rapid relaxation, paced breathing, and maintaining external focus as coping skills to be used in the face of social anxiety cues in daily living.

9. Review use the of calming and coping skills, reinforcing success and redirecting for failure.

Calming and Coping Skills Review Test Questions

1. In the treatment of SAD the technique of employing *rapid relaxation* in situations where social anxiety is likely to occur is a key practice in which of the following?

   A. Applied relaxation
   B. Cognitive restructuring
   C. Exposure therapy
   D. Progressive muscle relaxation
   Answer: A

2. Attentional refocusing to help manage social anxiety in social situations involves:

   A. Focusing on the external social task
   B. Focusing on one's internal self-talk
   C. Focusing on one's internal feeling state
   D. Focusing on repeating positive coping statements
   Answer: A

Talking Points

Discuss why attentional coping strategies would be used, in particular, with social anxiety.

- One of the processes thought to generate social anxiety and potentially interfere with the socially anxious person's ability to function in social situations is a focus of attention on anxious concerns, fears, and the like. This focus is thought not only to generate anxiety, but also compete with attention that could be given to the social task and facilitate performance of the task. One of the goals in social situations is to stay off the internal self-conscious focus, and on the reasonable expectations of the social interaction.

- As a coping strategy, thought-stopping (silently but assertively saying to oneself the word "stop") is used to halt the internal anxious train of thought.

- Attentional refocusing (changing from an anxious internal focus on anxiety and doubt to an external focus on the requirements of the social task) is then used to turn the focus of attention externally on the task at hand.
- In short, attentional strategies are intended to reduce anxiety and facilitate social functioning by focusing attention on the requirements of the social task, rather than on distracting, anxiety producing concerns.

Cognitive Restructuring

Cognitive restructuring helps the client understand the connection between fearful thoughts and the social anxiety and avoidance they produce. It helps the client identify, challenge, and change fearful appraisals to more realistic, less anxiety-provoking alternatives.

Several techniques are used in cognitive restructuring to facilitate this change, including psychoeducation, rational disputation, and ultimately in-session and homework assignments, termed "behavioral experiments," in which the patient identifies, challenges, and changes fearful beliefs in the context of their everyday experience. A summary of the primary steps in the cognitive restructuring procedure follows:

1. Educate the client about how cognitive appraisals influence emotional reactions.
2. Explain the rationale for cognitive restructuring: To change their perception of threat based on negatively biased predictions to predictions that are more in line with likely outcomes.
3. Identify, through self-monitoring and in-session discussion, the distorted self-talk.
4. Identify biases and generate reality-based alternatives that correct for the biases.
5. Convert the biased and alternative thoughts into predictions that can be tested through homework exposures (or "behavioral experiments").
6. Assign as homework the behavioral experiments or exposures.
7. Review, toward the goal of testing fearful predictions against healthy alternatives.
8. Reinforce the client's shift from distorted, negative self-talk to more positive, adaptive self-talk.
9. Make and reinforce the connection between positive thought changes and increased sense of calm and control.

The overarching goal of cognitive restructuring is to help the client shift from those biased, fear-based appraisals of threat (such as ones that overestimate the

Table 5.4   Cognitive Restructuring Objective and Interventions

Objective	Interventions
7. Identify, challenge, and replace biased, fearful self-talk with reality-based, positive self-talk.	1. Explore the client's schema and self-talk that mediates their social fear response; challenge the biases; assist him/her in generating appraisals that correct for the biases; and build confidence. 2. Assign the client to read about cognitive restructuring in books or treatment manuals on social anxiety. 3. Assign the client a homework exercise in which he/she identifies fearful self-talk, creates reality-based alternatives, and tests them in a chosen situation; review and reinforce success, providing corrective feedback for toward the goal of improvement.

likelihood of feared outcome and underestimate one's capacity to accomplish and manage realistic challenges) to alternatives that are more in line with likely outcomes.

Table 5.4 contains an objective and interventions that show how cognitive restructuring can be described in a treatment plan for social anxiety disorder.

Demonstration Vignette

Cognitive Restructuring

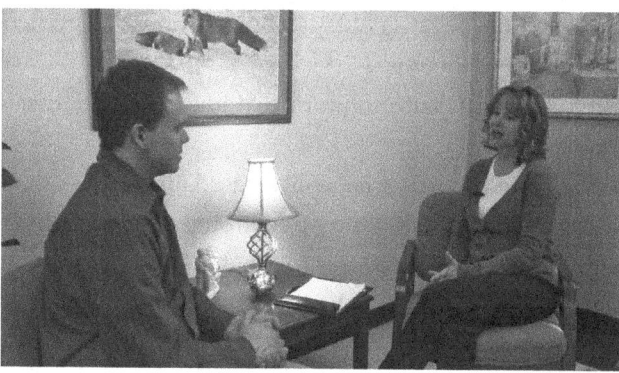

Here we present the transcript of the dialogue depicted in the cognitive therapy vignette.

Therapist: In previous sessions we've talked about how your self-talk triggers your emotions. We've also identified some of the self-talk that contributes to your anxiety before and during social situations. Do you recall some of those?

Client: Yes, and now that I'm aware of it, I see that I do it a lot.

Therapist: Okay, that's not surprising. So what have you noticed that you're saying to yourself?

Client: I say that I'm not going to be able to do this. I'm going to get too nervous. Everybody's going to notice. They're going to think something's wrong with me.

Therapist: Okay. And does it make sense to you that when you see the situation that way, it looks very scary and you don't feel confident at all?

Client: Yes. I feel I'm not going to be able to handle it and everyone will notice.

Therapist: And the self-talk makes you feel … ?

Client: It makes me feel bad and nervous and pretty scared usually.

Therapist: Sure. Now we also said that if we turn the self-talk into a prediction of what will happen, that it doesn't always line up with what actually happens. Your prediction usually overestimates these bad things and underestimates your ability to manage the situation. Do you remember that?

Client: Yeah, I can see these things don't happen like I thought they would. I just can't stop myself from thinking this way when I'm there.

Therapist: Well, that's normal. That's the way it usually works, unfortunately. And that's why just understanding it isn't enough. We want to challenge the self-talk directly. We want to prove it's telling the truth, and if not, we want to start dismissing it.

Client: Well, that makes sense. I just hope I can do it.

Therapist: You're willing to try then?

Client: I'll give it a try.

Therapist: All right. Now we've said that if the self-talk is overestimating the bad things, then there must be an alternative prediction that doesn't. One that's closer to what is likely to happen. Do you remember generating those alternative predictions?

Client: Yeah. Basically we said that I might get nervous, but if I stay focused on what I want to do, I can probably do it.

Therapist: Right. If losing control and not being able to do it is an overestimation, then a more realistic prediction is that you might have some anxiety, but you won't lose control. And if the self-talk underestimates your abilities to handle what you want to do, then an alternative prediction would be that you will manage the situation, even if you have to do it while you're nervous.

Client: Which I know is probably the case. It's just hard to believe when I'm in the situation.

Therapist: Right. The idea here is that is it more likely to become believable as you continue to test these predictions directly and see in your experience that you can believe the alternatives.

Client: I can see that.

Therapist: Okay, so let's find a situation where we can do this. We'll identify the predictions that you might have in fearful situations and the alternatives that are more realistic. Then we can plan out the situation, figure out what you want to do, and then go for it. In the next session we will go over how it turned out, and build from there. Does that sound okay?

Client: It sounds great.

Therapist: Okay, so what are some situations coming up this week where you might be able to practice?

Critique of the Cognitive Restructuring Demonstration Vignette

The following points were made in the critique:

➤ The vignette provides a good demonstration of various steps in cognitive restructuring: connecting thoughts to emotions, identifying biased thinking, developing alternative thoughts, rehearsal/homework, etc.

➤ Psychoeducation is an important component of cognitive restructuring.

➤ Understanding alone does not change feelings; there must be experiencing of alternative thoughts as accurate through homework (behavioral experiments).

➤ Group treatment is often used, as it acts as an exposure experience while using the restructuring process.

Additional points that could be made:

➤ The therapist needs to anticipate that the client will still feel anxious in spite of understanding the need to change thinking; using rehearsal, modeling and small steps toward facing situations will help.

➤ This process of teaching cognitive restructuring can take several sessions; this demonstration is moving very fast.

➤ This application is highly didactic. It's possible that she could accomplish these same goals through other, more interactive, means.

Comments you would like to make:

_____

_____

_____

Homework: The assignment "Journal and Replace Self-Defeating Thoughts" is an example of an exercise that is consistent with cognitive therapy and designed to help the client identify fearful self-talk and create reality-based, positive alternatives. The exercises "Negative Thoughts Trigger Negative Feelings" and "Journal of Distorted, Negative Thoughts" are examples of exercises designed to help the client make the connection between distorted thinking patterns and anxious emotions. These assignments also provide opportunity for the client to examine his thinking in response to events in her life and begin to develop positive, reality-based replacement thoughts. An exercise designed to help the client increase the frequency of positive thinking and talking about his capabilities, the world, and his future can be found in "Positive Self-Talk." The exercise "Restoring Socialization Comfort" is designed to assist the client in cognitive restructuring of specifically dysfunctional social anxiety messages (see www.wiley.com/go/anxietywb).

Cognitive Restructuring Review

1. What are the primary steps used in cognitive restructuring?

SUMMARY OF THE PRIMARY STEPS IN THE COGNITIVE RESTRUCTURING PROCEDURE

1. Educate the client about how cognitive appraisals influence emotional reactions.
2. Explain the rationale for cognitive restructuring: To change their perception of threat based on negatively biased predictions to predictions that are more in line with likely outcomes.
3. Identify, through self-monitoring and in-session discussion, the distorted self-talk.
4. Identify biases and generate reality-based alternatives that correct for the biases.
5. Convert the biased and alternative thoughts into predictions that can be tested through homework exposures (or "behavioral experiments").
6. Assign as homework the behavioral experiments or exposures.
7. Review, toward the goal of testing fearful predictions against healthy alternatives.
8. Reinforce the client's shift from distorted, negative self-talk to more positive, adaptive self-talk.
9. Make and reinforce the connection between positive thought changes and increased sense of calm and control.

Cognitive Restructuring Review Test Questions

1. Through discussions with his therapist, Tom comes to understand that his social anxiety escalates when thinking about the potentially embarrassing things that could happen to him in social situations. This represents what process in cognitive therapy?

   A. Identifying the connection between thought and emotion
   B. Identifying the biases contained in self-talk
   C. Monitoring self-talk
   D. Shifting from biased to alternative beliefs and predictions
   Answer: A

2. Once a client and therapist reach an understanding that the client's social fears contain biases that fuel anxiety and increase the urge to avoid, the next step in cognitive therapy is typically to:

   A. Assign behavioral experiment homework to help reinforce more reality-based appraisals
   B. Assist the client in generating reality-based alternatives that correct for the biases

    C. Explore early relationships that might be the source of these biased beliefs

    D. Teach the connection between thoughts and feelings

Answer: B

Talking Points

Although discussion and rational disputation of cognitive biases is a typical part of cognitive restructuring, it also involves exercises in which the client "tests" biased predictions against alternatives. Discuss why having the client test predictions in his or her own experience appears more effective in facilitating change than in-session discussion and disputation only.

This discussion could involve several possible factors. Consider the following:

- Intellectual understanding of the "unreasonableness" of phobic fears is a common feature in those who suffer from them, but it is not sufficient by itself to decrease the fear.

- On a similar note, phobic fears are to some degree "state dependent," meaning that the fears and urges to avoid are to some degree bound to the situation and typically take precedence in the client's response, regardless of how insightful the client is about its "unreasonableness" outside the situation.

- Experiential learning may be more convincing and enduring than intellectual understanding.

- Extinction of learned fears is more effective when done live ("in vivo") than in the imagination.

- Believability of alternative predictions may be best facilitated through actual experience than intellectual appreciation.

- Others

Situational Exposure

Exposure to situations in which the client fears social performance or interaction is a principle of ESTs for social anxiety. The avoidance that the socially anxious client engages in precludes opportunities to learn that these activities can be tolerated, that the anxiety will reduce to manageable levels, and that the feared outcomes often do not come true or are not as terrible or unmanageable as imagined. Accordingly, exposure encourages the client to re-enter feared social situations.

Exposure typically begins with the construction of a hierarchy of feared social activities that will guide the client through exposure exercises, ranging from lesser feared to greater feared situations. The selection of situations for actual exposure begins with those that are only mildly anxiety-provoking and builds up to the most feared encounters.

In the treatment of social anxiety, these exposures are typically practiced in session, using role-play of analogous situations, until mastered sufficiently. They are then moved between session using real world activities, something known as exposure *in vivo.* As always, reading assignments to supplement therapeutic interventions may be used. A summary of the steps used in the situational exposure procedure follows:

1. Create a hierarchy of feared situations or steps within a feared situation.
2. Select initial mildly anxiety-provoking situations from the fear hierarchy.
3. Lay out a step-by-step exposure plan.
4. Rehearse and practice exposures in session, planning the desired steps for accomplishing the task—as well as ways to manage realistically foreseeable challenges—until the client feels he/she can try them outside of sessions.
5. Participate in and model initial *in vivo* exposures, if needed.
6. Ask the client to do the exposure between sessions, recording periodic SUDs ratings throughout the exercise as well as thoughts, feelings, and actions they experienced.
7. Repeat exposures, to the degree possible, toward the goal of doing the exposure without undue anxiety.
8. Review each exposure with the client, providing reinforcing feedback for improving mastery.
9. Continue repeating and reviewing exposures until client confidence in doing them is restored.

The goals of social exposure are to build skills in managing social tasks without debilitating anxiety; build confidence and a sense of self efficacy in social situations; test predictions and shift from threatening to more reassuring appraisals of social situations and one's capacity to manage them; and extinguish anxiety (within and between session extinction). Table 5.5 contains an objective and interventions that show how situational exposure can be described in a treatment plan for social anxiety disorder.

Table 5.5   Situational Exposure Objective and Interventions

Objective	Interventions
8. Participate in gradual repeated exposure to feared social situations within individual or group therapy sessions; review with therapist.	1. Direct and assist the client in the construction of a hierarchy of feared situations associated with the social anxiety. 2. Select initial role-played exposures that have a high likelihood of being a successful experience for the client; do cognitive restructuring within and after the exposure; use behavioral strategies (e.g., modeling, rehearsal, social reinforcement) to facilitate successful completion of the exposure task; review with the client and group members, if done in group. 3. Assign the client to read about exposure in books or treatment manuals on social anxiety.
9. Undergo gradual repeated exposure to feared social situations outside of individual or group therapy sessions.	1. Assign the client homework exercises in which he/she does exposure exercises and records responses; review and reinforce success, providing corrective feedback toward improvement.

Demonstration Vignette

Situational Exposure for Social Anxiety

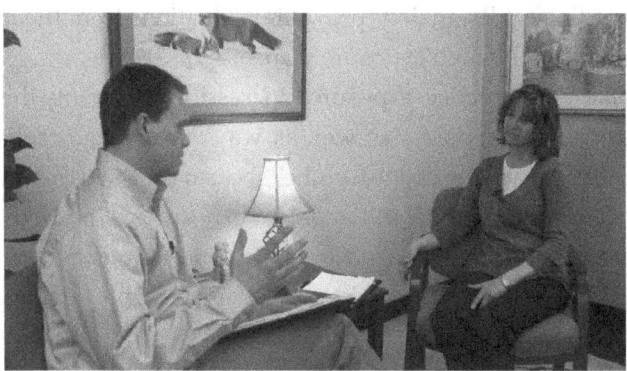

Here we present the transcript of the dialogue depicted in the situational exposure vignette.

[Therapist picks up following a review of a previous exposure]

Therapist: Well, would you agree that your exposure turned out well?

Client: Yes, I'd say it went very well.

Therapist: So what are you finding was most helpful?

Client: Well, laying them out, rehearsing them, that helps. Staying focused, not getting distracted by my heart rate, but I haven't been too anxious, either. Of course, I've been doing situations that are only 2s and 3s.

Therapist: Well, I think you may find that the things that have worked for 2s and 3s will also be helpful and effective as you tackle the higher levels. I think you've done very well. Do you feel like taking the next step?

Client: Well, I have that presentation to the board in a few weeks, so yeah.

Therapist: Right, and what did you rate that?

Client: I rated that a 5.

Therapist: So would you like to try?

Client: I think I need to.

Therapist: Okay. Let's start with what you want to do in this presentation to the Board. We'll lay out a plan. If you can write out what you want to say between this session and our next one and practice it, we can get it down the way you want.

Client: Sounds good.

Therapist: So, let's lay out what this presentation involves, and let's discuss how you would like it to go.

Client: Well, it is a sales summary presentation. It takes about five minutes. What I do is present the sales statistics for the last quarter . . . [fade out]

[Fade in to the next session where the client is going to practice the talk with the therapist]

Therapist: Okay, so you have the presentation?

Client: Yes, I do. I have it right here, as a matter of fact. I've practiced it at home.

Therapist: That's great. So like we've done before, I'm the audience and just act like you're at the meeting. I'll be asking for your SUD rating periodically, but just give it to me quickly and get right back on track. Remember how we've done that?

Client: Yeah, I remember that.

Therapist: So one of our goals is that no matter what happens—your heart races or you notice someone yawning or whatever it is, that you stay as focused as possible on what you're there to do. You want to act like you belong there. Remember, you're the one who knows this information, and your role is to convey it to the board so they can use it.

Client: Okay, I think I'm ready.

Therapist: One last thing—what's your rating right now?

Client: Right now it's about a 6.

Therapist: Okay. Are you ready to start?

Client: Okay, all right. [Pauses, then begins presentation] "Good morning. I'm [name] from accounting. I'm here to present the sales summaries for the quarter ending September . . . "

Critique of the Situational Exposure Demonstration Vignette

The following points were made in the critique:

➤ The therapist could have broken down the previous exposure experience that the client reported on at the outset.

➤ The vignette displayed a good use of homework in assigning preparation of the speech and practicing it before the next session.

➤ Good use of rehearsal, but future exposure could include more elements of the feared situation to mimic the real one (e.g., stand up, use a podium, put notes on a table, etc.).

➤ SUDs are used to assess anxiety level at frequent points in the exposure and rehearsal process; also serves to demonstrate to the client that he can function even when feeling some anxiety.

Additional points that could be made:

➤ Group treatment could be very powerful with this problem, using group members as "the board" audience.

➤ Role-played exposure could act out several different scenarios (e.g., questions are asked by board members, interruptions occur, lose your place for a moment, etc.).

Comments you would like to make:

_____

_____

_____

Homework: "Gradually Reducing Your Phobic Fear" is an example of an exercise that helps structure the development of the hierarchy of fear situations if used in session with the therapist (see www.wiley.com/go/anxietywb).

Situational Exposure Review

1. What are the primary steps involved in situational social exposure?

SUMMARY OF PRIMARY STEPS IN THE SITUATIONAL SOCIAL EXPOSURE PROCEDURE
1. Create a hierarchy of feared situations or steps within a feared situation.
2. Select initial mildly anxiety-provoking situations from the fear hierarchy.
3. Lay out a step-by-step exposure plan.
4. Rehearse and practice exposures in session, planning the desired steps for accomplishing the task—as well as ways to manage realistically foreseeable challenges—until the client feels he/she can try them outside of sessions.
5. Participate in and model initial _in vivo_ exposures, if needed.
6. Ask the client to do the exposure between sessions, recording periodic SUDs ratings throughout the exercise as well as thoughts, feelings, and actions they experienced.
7. Repeat exposures, to the degree possible, toward the goal of doing the exposure without undue anxiety.
8. Review each exposure with the client, providing reinforcing feedback for improving mastery.
9. Continue repeating and reviewing exposures until client confidence in doing them is restored.

---

2. What are common goals of situational social exposure?

GOALS OF SITUATIONAL EXPOSURE
- To build skills in managing social tasks without debilitating anxiety
- To build confidence and a sense of self-efficacy in social situations
- To test predictions and shift from threatening to more reassuring appraisals of social situations and one's capacity to manage them
- To extinguish anxiety (within and between session extinction)

Situational Exposure Review Test Questions

1. One of the first client objectives in situational exposure is to:

    A. Identify what is feared and at what level

    B. Identify self-talk that is associated with anxiety

    C. Lay out a step-by-step plan for the first exposure

    D. Learn strategies for coping with anxiety

    Answer: A

2. In situational exposure therapy for social anxiety, initial exposures are typically conducted:

    A. After the client has completed progressive muscle relaxation

    B. Live, in actual social situations

    C. Within therapy sessions, simulating social situations

    D. Without the assistance of the therapist

    Answer: C

Talking Points

Discuss possible mechanisms of action for exposure. This can be prompted by asking that question directly, or by asking an indirect question such as this: "What do you think the client experiences/learns through the course of exposure therapy that reduces their social fears and avoidance of situations that provoke them?"

ANSWERS WILL OBVIOUSLY REFLECT THE CONCEPTUAL MODELS OF THE PARTICIPANTS. EXAMPLES MAY INCLUDE

- Skills for managing social tasks effectively
- Confidence and a sense of self-efficacy in social situations
- Validation of alternative predictions that facilitate a shift in belief from threatening to more reassuring appraisals of social situations and one's capacity to manage them
- The extinction of conditioned anxiety
- Others

Social Skills Training

Some clients with social anxiety are actually very socially skilled. The problem is that the excessive anxiety they experience in social situations interferes with their ability to use these skills effectively. Others may lack the basic skills needed to initiate and maintain positive interpersonal interactions. For these individuals, social skills training is added to the treatment plan.

Social skills training is tailored to the individual's needs. It typically involves identification of the skill needed, education about the deficient skill and its appropriate use, therapist modeling, and repeated practice and review inside and outside of session. A summary of the social skills training procedure follows:

1. Explain the rationale for social skills training (e.g., to improve the predictability and controllability of social interaction, increase comfort, decrease uncertainty and anxiety).
2. Identify the skills needed to accomplish relevant social tasks (e.g., conversational skills, public speaking skills, assertive communication)
3. Provide psychoeducation about the skill needed.
4. Model and role-play interactions using skills.
5. Repeatedly practice, in and outside of sessions.
6. Review skill use, reinforcing success and redirecting for failure, toward the goal of developing adequate skills.

Table 5.6 contains an objective and interventions that show how social skills training can be described in a treatment plan for social anxiety disorder.

Table 5.6 Social Skills Training Objective and Interventions

Objective	Interventions
10. Learn and implement social skills to reduce anxiety and build confidence in social interactions.	1. Use instruction, modeling, and role-playing to build the client's general social and/or communication skills. 2. Assign the client to read about general social and/or communication skills in books or treatment manuals on building social skills.

Demonstration Vignette

Social Skills Training

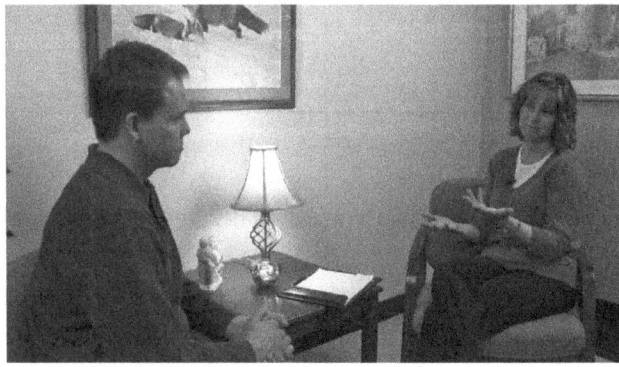

Here we present the transcript of the dialogue depicted in the social skills training vignette.

Therapist:	So, Bob, tell me what it's like for you to meet someone new—say, the husband of a colleague at a business dinner.
Client:	Well, I'll tell you, I'm usually a wreck ... I don't know what to say, and the more nervous I get, the harder it is to make conversation.
Therapist:	You know, lots of people don't learn simple social skills because they avoid social situations, so they don't have the opportunity to practice just basic conversation. How about if we do some role-play so you can get comfortable with it?
Client:	Okay, I'll give it a try.
Therapist:	All right. Now in your reading assignment, there were some guidelines to follow. I'd like to review those with you.
	The first one is for you to take the initiative to break the ice and greet the other person with just a simple, "Hi. How are you? I'm Bob."
	Second, you want to always have a follow-up question in mind for use after the introduction, something like, "Have you eaten at this restaurant before?"
	Third, be aware of your facial expression and remember—a smile is always a welcoming gesture.
	Next, you want to maintain eye contact for comfortable periods and be careful not to always look down or away.
	The fifth one is to watch your body language. Stay relaxed and lean toward people when talking or listening to them.
	Also, be mindful of people's names, and use their name in conversation to help you remember it and to make personal contact.
	Any finally, show interest in others by asking questions about their lives. I want you to avoid just talking about yourself.
Client:	I remember reading all those, I just wish I could do all of them.
Therapist:	That's why we're here. We're just here to practice it and practice it, and then you can try it at home and then with others as you get more familiar with it. So I want you to just try it out on me, and let's pretend that I'm the husband of one of your colleagues. You try out the guidelines, okay?
Client:	Okay, let's give it a try. "Hi. Is it Mike? I'm Bob Baker. It is good to meet you. Have you been here before?"

Critique of the Social Skills Training Demonstration Vignette

The following points were made in the critique:

➣ The educational component of skills training is shown.

➣ The rehearsal component is demonstrated well.

➣ The modeling component is missing; perhaps the skill level is high enough to make it unnecessary?

➣ Group treatment would be helpful and practical, using the feedback of members.

➣ This is a pretty socially skilled client, which raises the question as to whether anxiety reduction needs to be the focus rather than skill deficit reduction.

Additional points that could be made:

> ➤ Other social skills, such as assertiveness or public speaking, may be trained in this way.
> ➤ More components of real life could be included in the rehearsal (e.g., standing up to approach therapist, role-playing responses beyond introducing self, etc.).

Comments you would like to make:

_____

_____

_____

Homework: The homework assignments "Acknowledging My Strengths" and "What Are My Good Qualities" are example of interventions designed to build the client's confidence and awareness of positive skills and attributes (see www.wiley.com/go/anxietywb).

Social Skills Training Review

1. What are the primary steps involved in social skills training?

SUMMARY OF THE SOCIAL SKILLS TRAINING PROCEDURE
1. Explain the rationale for social skills training (e.g., to improve the predictability and controllability of social interaction, increase comfort, decrease uncertainty and anxiety).
2. Identify the skills needed to accomplish relevant social tasks (e.g., conversational skills, public speaking skills, assertive communication).
3. Provide psychoeducation about the skill needed.
4. Model and role-play interactions using skills.
5. Repeatedly practice, in and outside of sessions.
6. Review skill use, reinforcing success and redirecting for failure, toward the goal of developing adequate skills.

---

2. How does one decide whether to train social skills in the treatment of social anxiety disorder?

- As noted, some clients with social anxiety are actually very socially skilled. The problem is that the excessive anxiety they experience in social situations interferes with their ability to use these skills effectively. Others may lack the basic skills needed to initiate and maintain positive interpersonal interactions. For these individuals, social skills training is added to the treatment plan. Social skills training is tailored to the individual's needs, meaning that deficits in social skills that are important to the client's effective social functioning are targeted.

Social Skills Training Review Test Questions

1. A technique commonly used in social skills training, in which the therapists demonstrates the skill and its uses, is called:

    A. Assertiveness

    B. Modeling

    C. Rehearsal

    D. Exposure

    Answer: B

2. A practice common to social skills training, designed to facilitate the client's use of learned skills into day-to-day life, is:

    A. Self-monitoring to assess changes in mood

    B. Modeling of social skills by the therapist

    C. Reading assignments related to therapeutic topics

    D. Repeated practice by the client using homework and subsequent review

    Answer: D

Talking Points

As with learning any new, complex skill, reading or hearing about it is helpful, but seeing that skill modeled, practicing it, and shaping it through corrective feedback are important to acquiring and using it effectively. Consider a discussion with participants in which they compare their own clinical training to the training procedures used in social skills training.

Consider these questions to prompt the discussion:

- What are the parallels between the way we were trained clinically and the procedures commonly used in social skills training?
- What aspects of that training did you find most helpful in our own training?
- What implications do they have for the clinical practice of social skills training?

Other Common Approaches to Treatment

Therapists working with depression have also commonly used other approaches that may be part of an overall treatment plan. Examples include:

➤ Psychodynamic interventions exploring childhood criticism, abuse, abandonment, or other conflictual family situations

➤ Family/conjoint therapy to reinforce progress or reduce secondary gain

➤ Enhancing motivation through "stage of change" interventions

➤ Prescribing or referring for medication

Talking Points

What therapeutic approach(es) do you use for social anxiety and why?

- Ask participants what therapeutic approach or approaches they use with clients whose primary problem is social anxiety. Facilitate a discussion around the reasons for their choice.

- Common influences include professional training background, consistency of model with world-view, recent training in a new method, empirical evidence supporting the approach.

- Ask participants whether research support should or should not weigh heavily in the decision.

6

What Are Considerations for Relapse Prevention?

Chapter Review

1. What are the seven common considerations in relapse prevention?

COMMON CONSIDERATIONS IN RELAPSE PREVENTION
1. Explain the rationale of relapse prevention interventions.
2. Distinguish between lapse and relapse.
3. Identify high-risk situations for a lapse.
4. Review the application of skills learned in therapy to high-risk situations.
5. Encourage routine use of skills learned in therapy.
6. Consider developing a *coping card*.
7. Schedule periodic "booster" therapy sessions.

Chapter Review Test Question

1. John and his therapist identify previously feared situations that John plans to incorporate into his day-to-day activities after he leaves formal therapy. Which consideration in relapse prevention is being used in this example?

    A. Developing a coping card
    B. Distinguishing between lapse and relapse
    C. Encouraging routine use of skills learned in therapy
    D. Identifying high-risk situations for a lapse
    Answer: D

--- **Talking Point** ---

Select an example from the list of "Common Considerations in Relapse Prevention" and ask participants, "Why would this be important in helping a client prevent relapse?"

• The *Companion Workbook* contains several considerations.

Closing Remarks and Resources

As we note on the DVD, it is important to be aware that the research support for any particular empirically supported treatment (EST) supports the identified treatment as it was delivered in the studies supporting it. The use of only selected objectives or interventions from ESTs may not be empirically supported.

If you want to incorporate an EST into your treatment plan, it should reflect the major objectives and interventions of the approach. Note that in addition to their primary objectives and interventions, many ESTs have options within them that may or may not be used depending on the client's need (e.g., skills training).

Most treatment manuals, books, and other training programs identify the primary objectives and interventions used in the EST. Of course, in accordance with ethical guidelines, therapists should have competency in the services they deliver.

An existing resource for integrating research-supported treatments into treatment planning is the Practice*Planner*® series[1] of *Treatment Planners*. The series contains several books that have integrated goals, objectives, and interventions consistent with those of identified ESTs into treatment plans for several applicable problems and disorders:

➤ *The Severe and Persistent Mental Illness Treatment Planner* (Berghuis, Jongsma, & Bruce).
➤ *The Family Therapy Treatment Planner* (Dattilio, Jongsma, & Davis)
➤ *The Complete Adult Psychotherapy Treatment Planner* (Jongsma, Peterson, & Bruce)

---

[1] These books are updated frequently, check with the publisher for the latest editions, and information about the Practice*Planner*® series.

➤ *The Adolescent Psychotherapy Treatment Planner* (Jongsma, Peterson, McInnis, & Bruce).

➤ *The Child Psychotherapy Treatment Planner* (Jongsma, Peterson, McInnis & Bruce).

➤ *The Veterans and Active Duty Military Psychotherapy Treatment Planner* (Moore & Jongsma)

➤ *The Addiction Treatment Planner* (Perkinson, Jongsma, & Bruce)

➤ *The Couples Psychotherapy Treatment Planner* (O'Leary, Heyman, & Jongsma)

Finally, it is important to remember that the purpose of this series is to demonstrate the process of empirically informed psychotherapy treatment planning for common mental health problems. It is designed to be informational in nature and does not intend to be a substitute for clinical training in the interventions discussed and demonstrated. Of course, in accordance with ethical guidelines, therapists should have competency in the services they deliver.

A

Chapter Review Test Question Answers Explained

Chapter 1: What Are the DSM Criteria for Social Anxiety Disorder?

1. What feature of SAD helps differentiate it from normal shyness?

   A. SAD may involve anxiety symptoms: shyness typically does not.

   B. SAD may involve public speaking fears: shyness typically does not.

   C. SAD involves clinically significant distress or disability: shyness typically does not.

   D. SAD and shyness are two names for the same thing.

      A. *Incorrect*: Some shy individuals may experience signs (symptoms) of nervousness.

      B. *Incorrect*: Some shy individuals may fear and avoid public speaking.

      C. *Correct*: SAD is a clinical disorder, while shyness is not. Part of what defines SAD as a clinical disorder is the clinically significant distress or disability it causes.

      D. *Incorrect*: SAD is a clinical disorder as in C, above, while shyness is typically considered to be more of a personality feature that doesn't routinely result in clinically significant distress or disability.

2. Which of the following is most likely to be feared and avoided by someone with SAD?

   A. An interactive classroom

   B. Driving an automobile

   C. Flying in a plane

   D. Listening to a public speaker

      A. *Correct*: Situations in which the individual is likely to be subject to the scrutiny of others are commonly feared in SAD.

      B. *Incorrect*: Not the best answer, in part because it is not defined as a social situation. This fear is more common in agoraphobia and specific phobias.

C. *Incorrect*: Not the best answer in part because it is not defined as a social situation. This fear is more common in agoraphobia and specific phobias.

D. *Incorrect*: Although listening to speaker may be "sympathetically" anxiety-provoking for someone with SAD, being the speaker is usually more feared.

Chapter 2: What Are the Six Steps in Building a Treatment Plan?

1. A psychotherapy treatment plan can be drawn up without a diagnosis. For example, a good case formulation can be the basis of therapy. Why is it important to consider the diagnosis when developing a plan that could be informed by empirically supported treatments (ESTs)?

   A. A diagnosis is necessary to judge response to the EST.
   B. It is not necessary to consider diagnosis in empirically informed treatment planning.
   C. Some ESTs were developed and studied using diagnosis as inclusion criteria.
   D. Treatment may require medication, which typically requires diagnosis to be specified.
      A. *Incorrect*: Although diagnostic criteria can be used to assess response to treatment, outcome of treatment can be measured in other ways as well.
      B. *Incorrect*: See C.
      C. *Correct*: Many ESTs were developed for the treatment problems defined by a diagnosis. Knowing the diagnosis is particularly important in deciding whether an EST is applicable to a client.
      D. *Incorrect*: Although diagnosis is important in determining medication choice, this question pertains to ESTs, which are empirically supported psychological treatments.

2. The statement, "Identify, challenge, and change biased self-talk supportive of social anxiety" is an example of which of the following steps in a treatment plan?

   A. A primary problem
   B. A short-term objective
   C. A symptom manifestation
   D. A treatment intervention

    A. *Incorrect*: The primary problem (Step 1 in treatment planning) is the summary description, usually in diagnostic terms, of the client's primary problem.

    B. *Correct*: This is a short-term objective (Step 5 in treatment planning). It describes the desired actions of the client in the treatment plan.

    C. *Incorrect*: Symptom manifestations (Step 2 in treatment planning) describe the client's particular expression (i.e., manifestations or symptoms) of a problem.

    D. *Incorrect*: A treatment intervention (Step 6 in treatment planning) describes the therapist's actions designed to help the client achieve therapeutic objectives.

Chapter 3: What Is the Brief History of the Empirically Supported Treatments Movement?

1. Which statement best describes the process used to identify empirically supported treatments (ESTs)?

    A. Consumers of mental health services nominated therapies.

    B. Experts came to a consensus based on their experiences with the treatments.

    C. Researchers submitted their works.

    D. Task groups reviewed the literature using clearly defined selection criteria for ESTs.

        A. *Incorrect*: Mental health professionals selected ESTs.

        B. *Incorrect*: Expert consensus was not the method used to identify ESTs.

        C. *Incorrect*: Empirical works in the existing literature were reviewed to identify ESTs.

        D. *Correct*: Review groups consisting of mental health professionals selected ESTs based on predetermined criteria.

2. Based on the differences in their criteria, in which of the following ways are *well-established* treatments different than those classified as *probably efficacious?*

    A. Only probably efficacious treatments allowed the use of single case design experiments.

    B. Only well-established treatments allowed studies comparing the treatment to a psychological placebo.

    C. Only well-established treatments required demonstration by at least two different, independent investigators or investigating teams.

    D. Only well-established treatments allowed studies comparing the treatment to a pill placebo.

        A. *Incorrect*: Both sets of criteria allowed use of single subject designs. "Well-Established" required a larger series than did "Probably Efficacious" (see II under Well-Established and III under Probably Efficacious).

        B. *Incorrect*: Studies using comparison to psychological placebos were acceptable in both sets of criteria (see IA under Well-Established and II under Probably Efficacious).

        C. *Correct*: One of the primary differences between treatments classified as well-established and those classified as probably efficacious is that well-established therapies have had their efficacy demonstrated by at least two different, independent investigators (see V under Well-Established).

        D. *Incorrect*: Studies using comparison to pill placebos were acceptable in both sets of criteria (see IA under Well-Established and II under Probably Efficacious).

Chapter 4: What Are the Identified Empirically Supported Treatments for Social Anxiety Disorder?

1. Which statement best characterizes the use of social skills training in CBT for SAD?

    A. It is a key feature of treatment for SAD and always trained.

    B. It is not a key feature of treatment for SAD and is not trained.

    C. It is trained depending upon an assessment of skill deficits.

    D. It is trained only if public speaking fears are evident.

        A. *Incorrect*: Social skills may not be trained if a social skill deficit is not evident.

        B. *Incorrect*: Social skills typically trained when a social skill deficit is evident.

        C. *Correct*: Social skills are typically trained when a social skill deficit is evident.

        D. *Incorrect*: Any of several social skills, not just public speaking, may be trained depending on the client's deficit(s).

2. In the treatment of SAD the practice of asking client to repeatedly engage in feared and/or avoided social activities is called:

A. Applied relaxation
B. Cognitive restructuring
C. Exposure
D. Psychoeducation

    A. *Incorrect*: Applied relaxation involves applying relaxation in anxiety-provoking situations.

    B. *Incorrect*: Although cognitive therapy often asks client to engage in feared situations to test fears, the practice does not define this therapy as it does in C.

    C. *Correct*: The behavioral therapy technique of exposure is captured by this definition.

    D. *Incorrect*: Psychoeducation typically refers to an information exchange between client and therapist.

Chapter 5: How Do You Integrate Empirically Supported Treatments into Treatment Planning?

Calming and Coping Skills

1. In the treatment of SAD the technique of employing "rapid relaxation" in situations where social anxiety is likely to occur is a key practice in which of the following:

A. Applied relaxation
B. Cognitive restructuring
C. Exposure therapy
D. Progressive muscle relaxation

    A. *Correct*: Applied relaxation involves applying relaxation in anxiety-provoking situations.

    B. *Incorrect*: Cognitive restructuring is focused on identifying and changing thought content and processes relating to the problem.

    C. *Incorrect*: Although exposure therapy asks the client to repeatedly engage in feared and/or avoided activities, it does not specifically apply relaxation during them.

    D. *Incorrect*: Although PMR is designed to invoke relaxation, applied relaxation converts PMR into rapid relaxation and applies it in anxiety-provoking situations.

2. Attentional refocusing to help manage social anxiety in social situations involves:

    A. Focusing on the external social task
    B. Focusing on one's internal self-talk
    C. Focusing on one's internal feeling state
    D. Focusing on repeating positive coping statements
        A. *Correct*: One goal of attentional refocusing is to keep attention "on task," and off of anxiety-provoking thoughts.
        B. *Incorrect*: Attentional refocusing aims to keep attention focused externally, "on task."
        C. *Incorrect*: Attentional refocusing aims to keep attention focused externally, "on task."
        D. *Incorrect*: Although this type of "self-talk" may be encouraged in therapy, it does not describe attentional refocusing.

Cognitive Restructuring

1. Through discussions with his therapist, Tom comes to understand that his social anxiety escalates when thinking about the potentially embarrassing things that could happen to him in social situations. This represents what process in cognitive therapy?

    A. Identifying the connection between thought and emotion
    B. Identifying the biases contained in self-talk
    C. Monitoring self-talk
    D. Shifting from biased to alternative beliefs and predictions
        A. *Correct*: The vignette describes a client learning how thoughts influence emotions.
        B. *Incorrect*: The vignette does not describe the biases evident in the anxiety-provoking thoughts.
        C. *Incorrect*: Monitoring is a recording of self-talk typically done by the client prior to demonstrating its connection to feelings, identifying biases in it, and testing it against alternatives.
        D. *Incorrect*: The vignette does not describe a shift in thinking or belief, only the connection between thoughts and feelings.

2. Once a client and therapist reach an understanding that the client's social fears contain biases that fuel anxiety and increase the urge to avoid, the next step in cognitive therapy is typically to:

    A. Assign behavioral experiment homework to help reinforce more reality-based appraisals

    B. Assist the client in generating reality-based alternatives that correct for the biases

    C. Explore early relationships that might be the source of these biased beliefs

    D. Teach the connection between thoughts and feelings

        A. *Incorrect*: This step typically follows that described in B.

        B. *Correct*: Challenging the identified biases by generating reality-based alternatives that correct for the biases is the typical next step in cognitive therapy approaches.

        C. *Incorrect*: Although cognitive therapist may explore these in some cases, they typically work with the here-and-now.

        D. *Incorrect*: This step in therapy typically precedes identifying biases.

Situational Exposure

1. One of the first client objectives in situational exposure is to

    A. Identify what is feared and at what level

    B. Identify self-talk that is associated with anxiety

    C. Lay out a step-by-step plan for the first exposure

    D. Learn strategies for coping with anxiety

        A. *Correct*: This is a common first (assessment) step in any exposure therapy and leads to construction of a fear hierarchy to guide future exposures.

        B. *Incorrect*: This is a feature of cognitive therapy.

        C. *Incorrect*: This step comes after the object and situations that are feared and avoided have been identified.

        D. *Incorrect*: When used in exposure, this step is usually done after the assessment of feared activities has been completed.

2. In situational exposure therapy for social anxiety, initial exposures are typically conducted:

    A. After the client has completed progressive muscle relaxation

    B. Live, in actual social situations

    C. Within therapy sessions, simulating social situations

    D. Without the assistance of the therapist

        A. *Incorrect*: PMR may or may not be used in exposure therapy.

        B. *Incorrect*: Analogue or role-played exposures typically precede exposures done in vivo (live).

        C. *Correct*: As a means of gradating exposures, initial exposures for social anxiety are often simulations of real social situations.

        D. *Incorrect*: It is more typically for initial exposures to be therapist-assisted, again as a means of gradating them.

Social Skills Training

1. A technique commonly used in social skills training, in which the therapist demonstrates the skill and its uses, is called:

    A. Assertiveness
    B. Modeling
    C. Rehearsal
    D. Exposure
       A. *Incorrect*: Assertiveness describes a type of communication skill commonly taught in the treatment of social anxiety
       B. *Correct*: Therapists often model the use of a skill as part of teaching it.
       C. *Incorrect*: Rehearsal refers to the client's "practice-use" of a skill prior to using it a natural setting.
       D. *Incorrect*: Although a therapist may model exposures, modeling refers to the demonstration of the action.

2. A practice common to social skills training, designed to facilitate the client's use of learned skills in day-to-day life, is:

    A. Self-monitoring to assess changes in mood
    B. Modeling of social skills by the therapist
    C. Reading assignments related to therapeutic topics
    D. Repeated practice using homework and subsequent review
       A. *Incorrect*: Self-monitoring is more of an assessment tool than an intervention designed to facilitate skill use in day-to-day life.
       B. *Incorrect*: Modeling is used more to train a skill than to facilitate its use in day-to-day life.
       C. *Incorrect*: While psychoeducation may facilitate skill development and use, it is not intended as a direct intervention designed to facilitate skill use in day-to-day life.
       D. *Correct*: Repeated practice, review, and feedback are the techniques used in the training of most skills to facilitate independent use in day-to-day life.

Chapter 6: What Are Considerations for Relapse Prevention?

1. John and his therapist identify situations that John fears could potentially set him back should he encounter one. They plan to review these encounters and develop a plan for coping with them. Which consideration in relapse prevention is being used in this example?

   A. Developing a coping card
   B. Distinguish between lapse and relapse
   C. Encouraging routine use of skills learned in therapy
   D. Identifying high-risk situations for a lapse
      A. *Incorrect*: This is a technique used by some clients to help them remember key therapeutic points and strategies outside of therapy.
      B. *Incorrect*: This is a psychoeducational intervention designed in part to help prevent misinterpretation of potentially manageable "setbacks" as an unmanageable relapse.
      C. *Incorrect*: This intervention is designed to transport skill use into every-day applications, not just ones that represent a higher risk for relapse.
      D. *Correct*: The vignette describes identifying high-risk situations. John and his therapist will then review and develop a plan for managing them.

STUDY PACKAGE
CONTINUING EDUCATION
CREDIT INFORMATION

Evidence-Based Treatment Planning for Social Anxiety Disorder

Our goal is to provide you with current, accurate and practical information from the most experienced and knowledgeable speakers and authors.

Listed below are the continuing education credit(s) currently available for this self-study package. *Please note: Your state licensing board dictates whether self study is an acceptable form of continuing education. Please refer to your state rules and regulations.*

COUNSELORS: PESI, LLC is recognized by the National Board for Certified Counselors to offer continuing education for National Certified Counselors. Provider #: 5896. We adhere to NBCC Continuing Education Guidelines. This self-study package qualifies for 1.75 contact hours.

SOCIAL WORKERS: PESI, LLC, 1030, is approved as a provider for continuing education by the Association of Social Work Boards, 400 South Ridge Parkway, Suite B, Culpeper, VA 22701. www.aswb.org. Social workers should contact their regulatory board to determine course approval. Course Level: All Levels. Social Workers will receive 1.75 (Clinical) continuing education clock hours for completing this self-study package.

PSYCHOLOGISTS: PESI, LLC is approved by the American Psychological Association to sponsor continuing education for psychologists. PESI, LLC maintains responsibility for these materials and their content. PESI is offering these self- study materials for 1.5 hours of continuing education credit.

ADDICTION COUNSELORS: PESI, LLC is a Provider approved by NAADAC Approved Education Provider Program. Provider #: 366. This self-study package qualifies for 2.0 contact hours.

MARRIAGE & FAMILY THERAPISTS: This activity consists of 1.75 clock hours of continuing education instruction. Credit requirements and approvals vary per state board regulations. Please save the course outline, the certificate of completion you receive from the activity and contact your state board or organization to determine specific filing requirements.

NURSES/NURSE PRACTITIONERS/CLINICAL NURSE SPECIALISTS: This independent study package meets the criteria for a formally approved American Nurses Credentialing Center (ANCC) Activity . PESI, LLC is an approved provider by the American Psychological Association, which is recognized by the ANCC for behavioral health related activities.

Nurses completing these learner-directed materials will earn 1.9 contact hours.

Procedures:

1. Review the workbook that contains the written materials.

2. Review and study the recording.

3. If seeking credit, the following must be completed on the post-test/evaluation form:

>   -Complete post test/evaluation in entirety; including your email address to
>   receive your certificate much faster versus by mail.
>   -Upon completion, mail to the address listed on the form, or fax to 1-800-554-
>   9775, "Attention: CE Dept".

Your completed post test/evaluation will be graded. If you receive a passing score (70% and above), you will be emailed/faxed/mailed a certificate of successful completion with earned continuing education credits. (Please write your email address on the post test/ evaluation form for fastest response.) If you do not pass the post-test, you will be sent a letter indicating areas of deficiency, and another post test to complete. The post-test must be resubmitted and receive a passing grade before credit can be awarded. We will allow you to re-take as many times as necessary to receive a certificate.

If you have any questions, please feel free to contact our customer service department at 1.800.844.8260.

Course Content

This Workbook is a supplement to the Evidence-Based Treatment Planning for So-cial Anxiety Disorder DVD, which is focused on informing mental health and addiction counselors about evidence-based psychological treatment. The content in the DVD and workbook will examine the following: DSM Criteria for Social Anxiety Disorder, Six Steps to a Treatment Plan, Introduction to ESTs for Social Anxiety Disorder, Integrating ESTs for Social Anxiety Disorder into Treatment Planning, Calming and Coping Skills, Cognitive Restructuring, Situational Exposure, Social Skills Training, Other Common Approaches to Treatment, and Relapse Prevention.

PESI LLC
PO BOX 1000
Eau Claire, WI 54702-1000

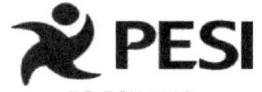

Evidence-Based Treatment Planning for Social Anxiety Disorder

PO BOX 1000
Eau Claire, WI 54702
800-844-8260

Any persons interested in receiving credit may photocopy this form, complete and return with a payment of $15.00 per person CE fee. A certificate of successful completion will be sent to you. To receive your certificate sooner than two weeks, rush processing is available for a fee of $10. Please attach check or include credit card information below.

Mail to: PESI, PO Box 1000, Eau Claire, WI 54702 or fax to PESI (800) 554-9775 (both sides)

CE Fee: $15: (Rush processing fee: $10)　　　　**Total to be charged** _____

Credit Card #: _____ **Exp Date:** _____ **V-Code*:** _____
(*MC/VISA/Discover: last 3-digit # on signature panel on back of card.) (*American Express: 4-digit # above account # on face of card.)

	LAST	FIRST	M.I.

Name (please print): _____　_____　_____

Address: _____ Daytime Phone: _____

City: _____ State: _____ Zip Code: _____

Signature: _____ Email: _____

Date Completed: _____ Actual time (# of hours) taken to complete this offering: _____hours

Program Objectives After completing this publication, I have been able to achieve these objectives:

Explain the process and criteria for diagnosing social anxiety disorder	Yes	No
List the six steps in building a psychotherapy treatment plan	Yes	No
Examine how empirically supported treatments for social anxiety have been identified	Yes	No
Examine the objectives and treatment interventions consistent with those of identified empirically supported treatments for social anxiety disorder	Yes	No
Describe how to construct a psychotherapy treatment plan and inform it with objectives and treatment interventions identified empirically supported treatments for social anxiety disorder	Yes	No
Identify common considerations in the prevention of relapse of social anxiety disorder	Yes	No

PESI LLC
PO BOX 1000
Eau Claire, WI 54702-1000

CE Release Date: 3/31/10

Participant Profile:
1. Job Title: _____ Employment setting: _____

1. Many people experience some level of anxiety in certain social situations (e.g., being interviewed, public speaking). Which of the following diagnostic criteria differentiates these common social anxieties from social anxiety disorder (SAD) as defined in psychiatric classification systems such as the DSM?
a. The fears and/or avoidance in SAD cause clinically significant distress, disability, or both.
b. The intensity of the physical symptoms in SAD is stronger than in normal social anxiety.
c. The number of social situations that are feared in SAD is more than with normal social anxiety.
d. There are far more physical symptoms in social anxiety disorder than in normal social anxiety.

2. Which of the following situations is most likely to be avoided by someone with SAD?
a. Being a passenger in a plane.
b. Being a spectator in a sports arena.
c. Being a member of a committee.
d. Being alone at home.

3. John's symptoms of social anxiety include fear of being scrutinized, situational panic attacks when he feels he is the center of attention, and avoidance of situations in which he must talk in front of other people. These features of social anxiety as manifested in John would be described under which of the following headings in a treatment plan?
a. Behavioral definitions.
b. Primary problem.
c. Short-term objectives.
d. Therapeutic interventions.

4. Cognitive and behavioral therapies are currently the only therapies that have met the APA Division 12's criteria for "well-established" in the treatment of social anxiety disorder?

TRUE   FALSE

5. ESTs for social anxiety disorder rarely ask the client to practice his/her feared social performances and other social interactions during or between therapy sessions.

TRUE   FALSE

6. Which of the following best describes the use of communication skills training in ESTs for social anxiety disorder (SAD)?
a. These skills are always trained in ESTs for SAD.
b. These skills are not trained in ESTs for SAD.
c. These skills are trained when panic attacks are a part of the clinical picture.
d. These skills are usually trained only when a skill deficit is evident.

7. John and his therapist discuss alternatives to John's interpretation that people who yawn while he is talking are bored with him. This type of intervention is consistent with which of the following treatment techniques used in ESTs for SAD?
a. Calming and coping skills training.
b. Cognitive restructuring.
c. Exposure.
d. Social skills training.

8. Which of the following statements from a treatment plan describes an example of a key intervention used in ESTs for social anxiety disorder?
a. "Explore possible childhood sexual abuse as a source for current social anxiety."
b. "Explore the client's early experiences with parental discipline as a possible source for current social anxiety."
c. "Explore unexpressed anger (anger turned inward) as a possible source for current social anxiety."
d. "Role-play with the client selected social scenarios about which the client is anxious."

9. Which of the following best describes objectives and interventions consistent with ESTs for social anxiety disorder noted in this program?
a. Applied relaxation, reassurance, stress management, cognitive restructuring, and relapse prevention.
b. Confrontation regarding avoidance, exploring abuse history, reviewing childhood conflicts.
c. Psychoeducation, calming and coping strategies, cognitive restructuring, exposure, and social skills training.
d. Supportive counseling, motivational interviewing, stress management, skills training, and relapse prevention.

10. A common consideration in relapse prevention noted in this program is to encourage the routine use of skills learned in therapy after therapy is over.

TRUE   FALSE

PESI LLC
PO BOX 1000
Eau Claire, WI 54702-1000